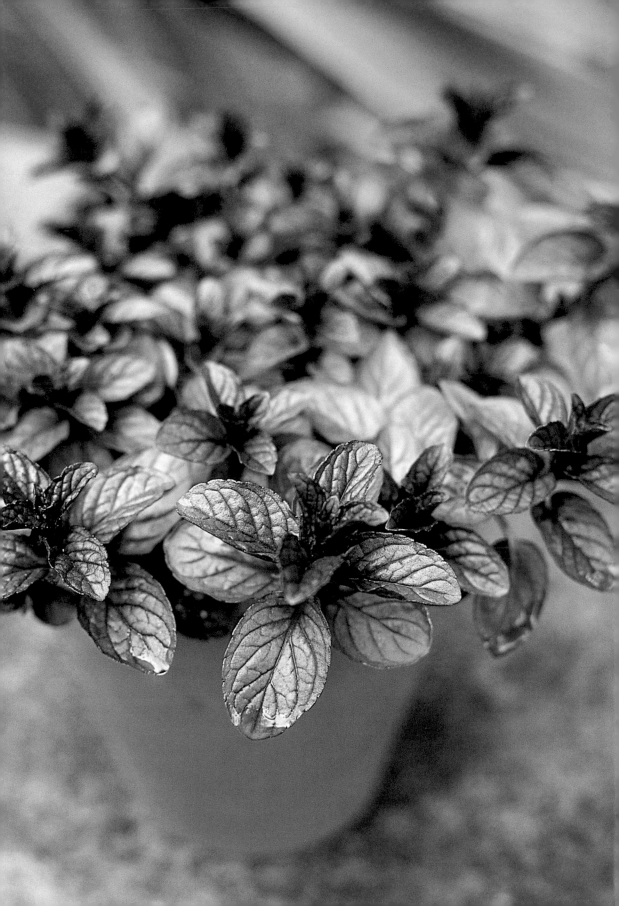

The
A~Z of
essential oils

What they are, where they come from, how they work

E. Joy Bowles

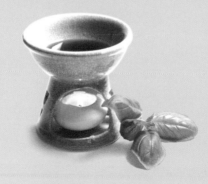

BARRON'S

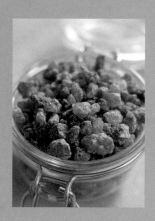

A QUARTO BOOK

First edition for the United States,
Canada, and the Philippine Republic
published in 2003
by Barron's Educational Series, Inc.

All inquiries should be addressed to:
Barron's Educational Series, Inc.
250 Wireless Boulevard
Hauppauge, NY 11788
http://www.barronseduc.com

International Standard Book Number
0-7641-5616-0
Library of Congress Catalog Card Number
2002107356

QUAR.OILS
Conceived, designed, and produced by
Quarto Publishing plc
The Old Brewery
6 Blundell Street
London N7 9BH

PROJECT EDITOR Paula McMahon
COPY EDITOR Mary Senechal
DESIGNERS Louise Clements, Katie Eke,
        Michelle Stamp
PHOTOGRAPHER Sarah Cuttle
PROOF READER Anna Bennett
INDEXER Pamela Ellis

ART DIRECTOR Moira Clinch
PUBLISHER Piers Spence

Manufactured by Universal Graphics,
Singapore
Printed by Midas Printing International
Limited, China

9 8 7 6 5 4 3 2 1

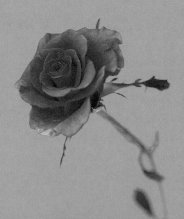

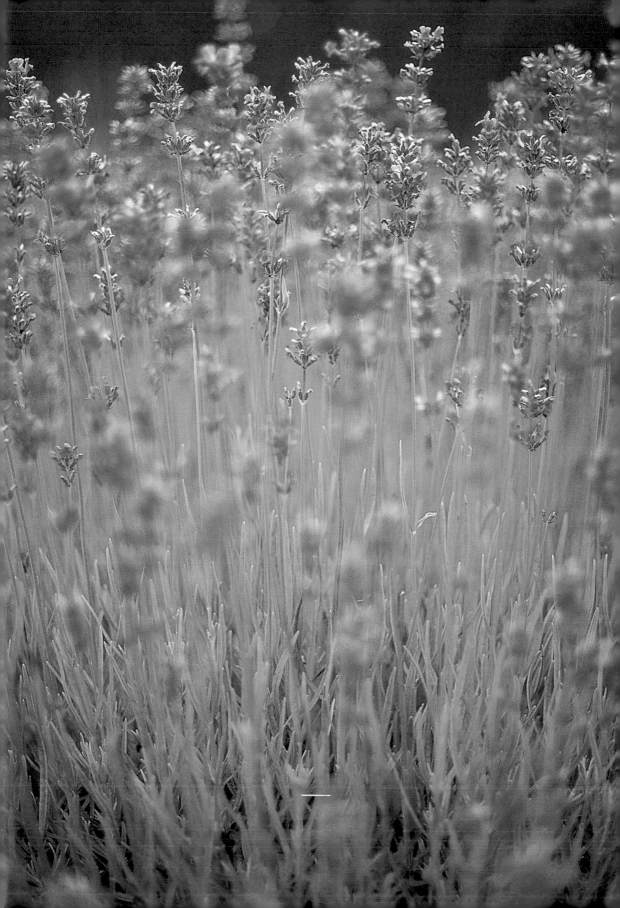

Contents

PREFACE 8

HOW TO USE THIS BOOK 9

SECTION 1

Aromatherapy oils:the essentials 10

Humans and fragrant plants 12

From plant to bottle 14

Tinctures to teas 16

The power of scent 22

Massage and essential oils 24

Temples and scalp 26

Face 27

Neck and shoulders 28

Back 30

Hands 32

Feet 33

Therapeutic properties of essential oils 34

Skin 36

Muscles 37

Germs and infections 38

Stress 39

SECTION 2

The directory of essential oils 40

Abies alba 42

Achillea millefolium 44

Angelica archangelica 46

Aniba rosaeodora 48

Anthemis nobilis, Chamaemelum nobile 50

Boswellia carterii 52

Cananga odorata var. *genuina* 54

Canarium luzonicum 56

Cardamomum elettaria 58

Citrus aurantium var. *amara* (flowers) 60

Citrus aurantium var. *amara* (leaves and twigs) 62

Citrus bergamia 64

Citrus latifolia 66

Citrus limonum 68

Citrus paradisii 70

Citrus reticulata, C. deliciosa 72

Citrus sinensis 74

Commiphora myrrha, C. molmol 76

Contents: Common name

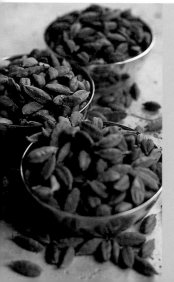

Angelica 46

Aniseed 130

Basil {Sweet Basil} 124

Bay Laurel {or Sweet Bay} 100

Benzoin 146

Bergamot 64

Black Pepper 134

Cajuput 110

Cardamom 58

Cedarwood, Virginia 98

Chamomile, Roman or English 50

Chamomile, German 106

Citronella 86

Clary sage 142

Coriander 78

Cypress 80

Elemi 56

Eucalyptus 88

Fir, White 42

Frankincense (Olibanum) 52

Geranium 128

Ginger 154

Grapefruit 70

Immortelle 92

Jasmine 94

Juniper 96

Lavender 102

Lavender, Spike 104

Lemon 68

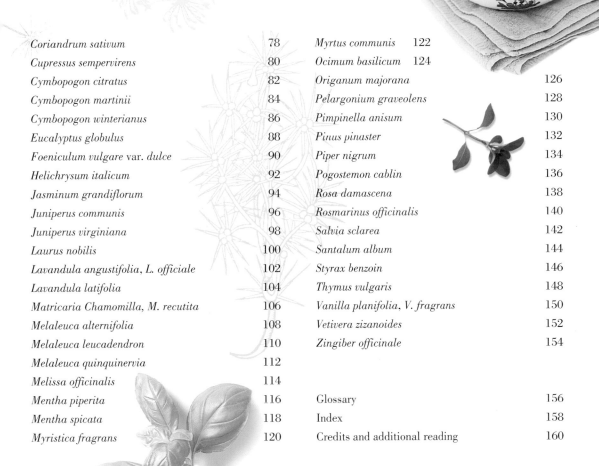

Coriandrum sativum 78
Cupressus sempervirens 80
Cymbopogon citratus 82
Cymbopogon martinii 84
Cymbopogon winterianus 86
Eucalyptus globulus 88
Foeniculum vulgare var. dulce 90
Helichrysum italicum 92
Jasminum grandiflorum 94
Juniperus communis 96
Juniperus virginiana 98
Laurus nobilis 100
Lavandula angustifolia, L. officiale 102
Lavandula latifolia 104
Matricaria Chamomilla, M. recutita 106
Melaleuca alternifolia 108
Melaleuca leucadendron 110
Melaleuca quinquinervia 112
Melissa officinalis 114
Mentha piperita 116
Mentha spicata 118
Myristica fragrans 120

Myrtus communis 122
Ocimum basilicum 124
Origanum majorana 126
Pelargonium graveolens 128
Pimpinella anisum 130
Pinus pinaster 132
Piper nigrum 134
Pogostemon cablin 136
Rosa damascena 138
Rosmarinus officinalis 140
Salvia sclarea 142
Santalum album 144
Styrax benzoin 146
Thymus vulgaris 148
Vanilla planifolia, V. fragrans 150
Vetivera zizanoides 152
Zingiber officinale 154

Glossary 156
Index 158
Credits and additional reading 160

Lemongrass 82
Lime 66
Mandarin 72
Melissa
   {or Lemon Balm} 114
Myrrh 76
Myrtle 122
Neroli 60
Niaouli 112
Nutmeg 120
Palmarosa 84

Patchouli 136
Peppermint 116
Petitgrain 62
Pine 132
Rose 138
Rosemary 140
Rosewood
   {or Bois-de-Rose} 48
Sandalwood 144
Spearmint 118
Sweet Fennel 90

Sweet marjoram 126
Sweet Orange 74
Tea tree
   {Australian} 108
Thyme
   {Sweet Thyme} 148
Vanilla 150
Vetiver 152
Yarrow 44
Ylang ylang 54

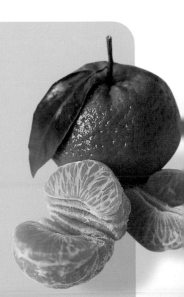

Preface

Aromatherapy is a complementary therapy that is coming of age. The power of fragrance has been known to humans since the dawn of time. Pleasant odors attract us—think of the scent of ripe strawberries on a summer's day, or the smell of a newborn baby. Equally, bad odors can cloud our mood or even make us feel physically sick.

Using the aromas of plants to promote a sense of well-being is a universal human activity. In many cultures, flowers are brought into the house to be appreciated for their beauty and scent. The use of perfumes enables us to be continually surrounded by aromas that please us. Fragrant incense made from plant materials is used in the rites of many religions to enhance the spiritual experience of the participants.

As humans evolved with sweet-smelling plants growing around them, they learned how to use plants and their extracts for curing disease as well as for pleasure. Essential oils are part of the herbal pharmacopeia (store of medicines and medical knowledge), and are proving to be potent, human-friendly alternatives to synthetic pharmaceuticals.

Growing up with fragrant plants

My childhood in Kenya was lived amid enticing scents. Our yard contained lemon verbena, honeysuckle, and roses, salvia with sweet honey in the flower tips, and spicy nasturtium leaves. A wattle tree oozed resinous sap, and a tall pine hedge vented its fragrance in the hot African sun. There were drooping pepper trees, a jacaranda with its sweet woody scent, and a custard-apple tree bearing spicy, succulent fruit. After the rains, the freesias bloomed, and the air carried the evanescent odor of violets.

Every week the fruit and vegetable man brought his fragrant cargo: ripe red plums at Christmas, tangerines, strawberries, several varieties of banana, pineapples, mangoes, pawpaws, guavas, lemons, oranges, red grapefruit, tomatoes, squashes, and rustly onions. Our yearly trips to the coast brought the sensual delights of cardamom, cumin, cinnamon bark, lime juice, freshly roasted cashew nuts, and passion fruit.

We moved to Australia, where I majored in biology and organic chemistry, and where a natural cosmetics course introduced me to the use of herbs and essential oils. A serendipitous meeting with an aromatherapy teacher in Sydney led to the design of a course in the chemistry of essential oils and to the marriage of my life's interests.

This "A–Z" aims to introduce you also to these wonderful fragrant substances, to their therapeutic properties, and to the ways in which they can enhance your life.

E. Joy Bowles

How to use this book

There are over 200 commercially available essential oils. Those selected for this book are used by nonmedical aromatherapists, and cover most conditions that can be safely treated with essential oils following the guidelines given. The oils are organized A to Z by the international system of botanical Latin names of the plants. Refer to the Contents page at the front of the book for a quick checklist of common English and Latin names for each plant.

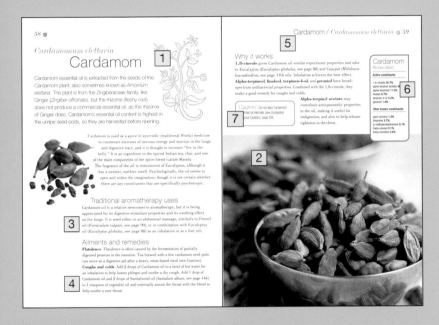

1. Latin and common names are given. Abbreviated names of botanists, which are often appended to Latin names (for example, L. for Linnaeus) have been avoided to prevent confusion.

2. Beautiful identification picture, usually of the plant part or product from which the oil is extracted.

3. Traditional use: For a fuller understanding, this section covers historical uses of the oil, or the herb from which the oil is extracted.

4. Ailments: Refer to this section to find out which ailments can be treated with the oil. Other authors may give alternative suggestions, but those selected are based on practical experience.

5. Why it works: Some essential-oil constituents have specific therapeutic activities. Significant constituents of each oil are listed, with brief descriptions of their contribution to the therapeutic activity of the oil.

6. Main active constituents/other constituents: Some constituents are active in small amounts, others in larger amounts. If listed in "Why it works," the constituents contribute to the oil's activities. Use this list to compare the composition of different oils.

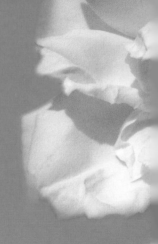

SECTION 1

aromatherapy oils : the essentials

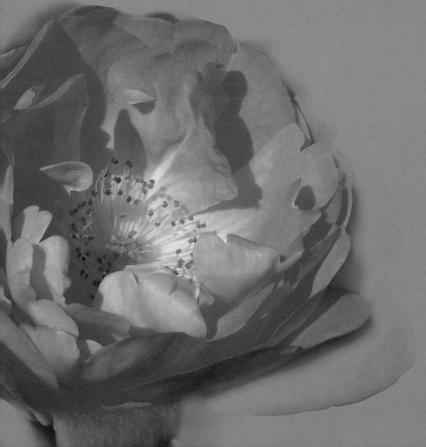

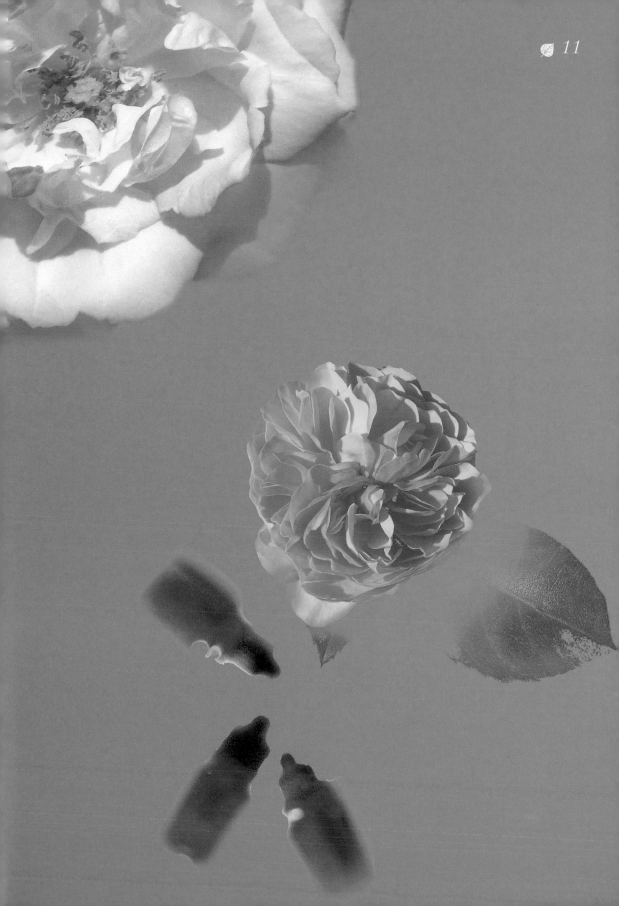

Humans and fragrant plants

Humans and scent ❧

The sense of smell in humans evolved to detect food and other environmental signals, such as smoke. Studies of human pheromones, the body odors produced by humans, show that perception of body odor can affect our choice of mate. Smells that we consider pleasant have a beneficial effect on our mood, whereas smells that seem disgusting can have a detrimental effect on our mood.

The olfactory nerve cells responsible for our sense of smell are located in the top of our nasal cavity. Each nerve cell has different receptors that can respond to different odor molecules. When an odor molecule fits into a receptor, an electrical message is sent to the brain. The olfactory information is processed by the limbic system, an area of the brain that initiates mood and memory formation. The links between odor and mood depend upon individual experience, but there are cultural and geographical odors that help frame our perception of the world, often without our conscious recognition.

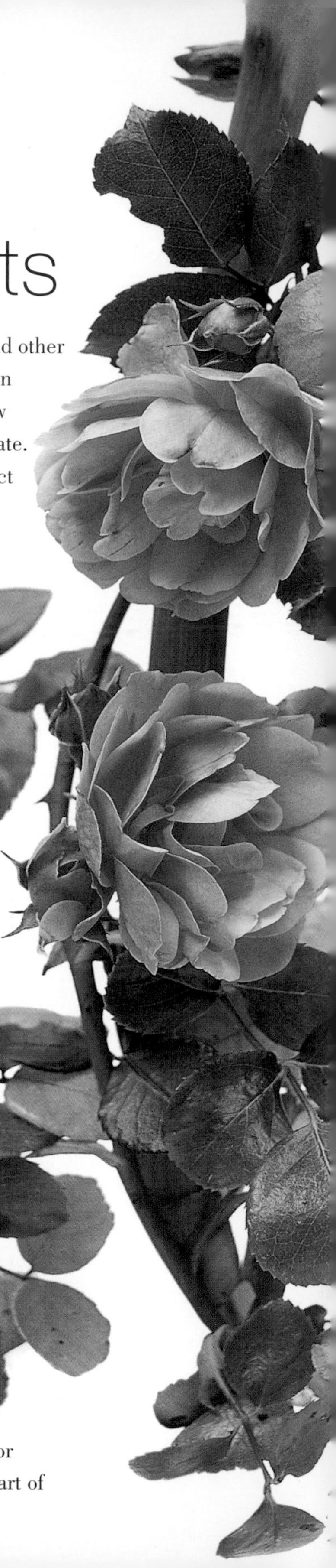

Evolving with plants ❧

Human fascination with fragrance must have started with our response to the aromas and odors of the natural world. Some flowers produce heady scents to attract pollinating insects. To defend themselves against predators and disease, other plants deploy a range of chemical defenses. Some plant chemicals, such as the juice from chili pods, cause extreme irritation; some are poisonous; others have a laxative or emetic effect; most taste bitter or pungent. Essential oils are part of

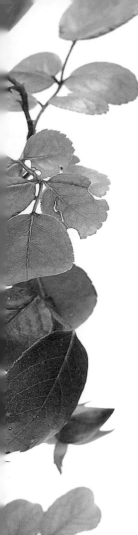

this chemical arsenal. Most of the essential oils found in leaves, rinds of fruit, and seeds deter insects and herbivores from eating them. Essential oils in the bark and heartwood of trees are probably a protection against fungal or bacterial infection. Humans have found ways of using these bioactive essential oils to deal with similar problems of defense against disease.

Humans have cultivated food and medicinal plants for many centuries. Aromatic plants have become an integral part of cuisine. In India, there is a medical tradition known as ayurveda, which means "the science of life." It is a holistic approach to the maintenance of wellness, using food, spices, herbs, exercise, and meditative practices to bring a person into a healthy balance. Ayurvedic cooking incorporates essential oil-bearing herbs and spices for their therapeutic effects.

> **Cooking, herbalism, and perfumery** 🌸

Similarly, Italians use rosemary, oregano, marjoram, thyme, and sage, which all contain essential oils. Research shows that essential oils from these herbs have antioxidant and antibacterial properties, making them natural preservatives, both for the food and the human body. Plant aromas are also associated with spiritual and mystical practices. From ancient times, essential oil-bearing woods and resins were burned in almost all cultures to give a pleasant-smelling smoke in religious ceremonies, as an offering to the gods. The fact that essential oils and other fragrant substances also bring pleasure to humans prompted the development of the perfumery industry.

In the history of the human search for wholeness, health, and happiness through aromatic plants, the essential oils are the major players. It is no surprise that aromatherapy is evolving as a therapy in its own right.

The term aromatherapy was first used in France in the 1930s, when Dr. Marguerite Maury began her health and beauty treatments with essential oils. In France, the beauty industry was always linked with health, and the use of the essential oils in beauty was a natural progression from their existing application in the French herbal medicine tradition. The oils were inhaled, ingested, and massaged onto the face and body, as required, but there was always the belief that the aroma was a significant component of the treatment.

> **Modern-day aromatherapy** 🌸

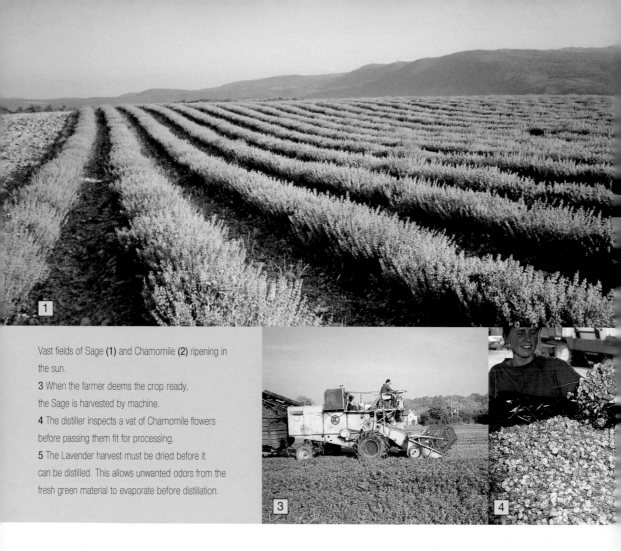

Vast fields of Sage **(1)** and Chamomile **(2)** ripening in the sun.

3 When the farmer deems the crop ready, the Sage is harvested by machine.

4 The distiller inspects a vat of Chamomile flowers before passing them fit for processing.

5 The Lavender harvest must be dried before it can be distilled. This allows unwanted odors from the fresh green material to evaporate before distillation.

From plant to bottle

The extraction of essential oils from plants was discovered by Persian and Egyptian alchemists. They boiled the aromatic plant material in a closed flask, allowed it to cool, and then collected the thin layer of essential oil floating on the surface of the water. Legend has it that a servant of Queen Cleopatra first noticed this fragrant essential oil film on one of the Queen's rose-petal baths.

Modern extraction processes are not so different, though better results are obtained by passing steam over the plant material rather than boiling it in water. A condensing pipe is used to cool the resulting vapor, and the essential oil can be collected off the surface of the resultant liquid. The waters of distillation are known as

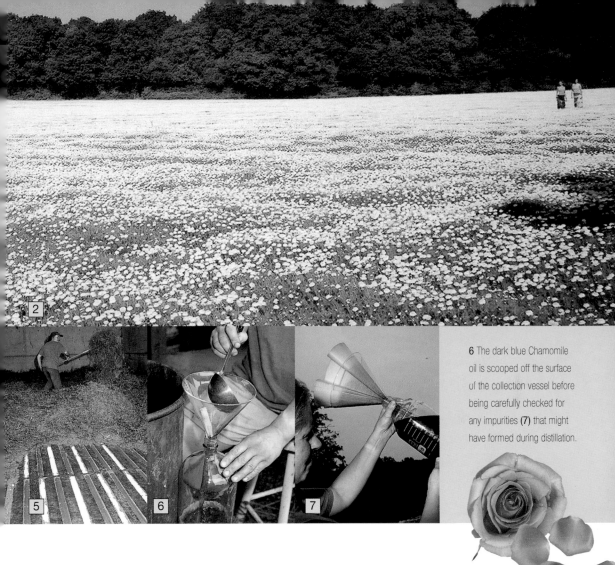

2

5

6

7

6 The dark blue Chamomile oil is scooped off the surface of the collection vessel before being carefully checked for any impurities **(7)** that might have formed during distillation.

Above: Rose petals cannot be harvested by machine and have to be picked by hand. This accounts for the relative expense of rose oil.

hydrosols or hydrolats, and contain aromatic water-soluble molecules. The rose water and orange flower water used in cookie making and confectionery are from the distillation process. Other hydrosols are being investigated for their antibacterial properties, as their acidic pH makes them active in this regard.

Essential oils can also be extracted with chemical solvents. The plant material can be crushed and left to sit in vegetable oil to produce an infused oil, which contains both essential oil and any vegetable oil from the plant itself. Citrus oils are usually extracted by squeezing the fruit peel between rollers in a process known as expression or cold pressing, but they can also be steam distilled.

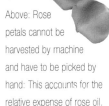

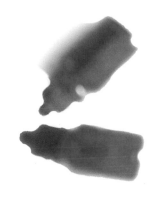

Tinctures to teas

<table>
<tr><td>

Other plant extracts
🌹

</td><td>

There are other types of plant extract that also contain essential oils, but they also contain other substances that give the extracts, because they have different therapeutic properties. These extracts are often available from essential-oil suppliers, so it is important to be aware of the difference.

</td></tr>
</table>

The first of these other plant extracts are the herbal tinctures. A tincture is made by putting the plant material into a mixture of water and 25% ethanol, and leaving it there for about two weeks. Tinctures contain essential oils and water-soluble compounds with different therapeutic properties from the essential oils. In some case tinctures can be used in the same way as essential oils, for example, Benzoin (see page 146), but in most cases they are not interchangeable.

Infused oils are made by covering the plant material with a vegetable oil and leaving it in the sun for about two weeks. The vegetable oil acts as a solvent, and extracts not only any essential oil compounds, but also fats, waxes, colored pigments, and other fat-soluble substances from the plant material. Infused oils can be used on their own as massage oils, or have other essential oils added to them. Examples of infused oils are Marigold (*Calendula officinalis*) and St. John's Wort (*Hypericum perforatum*), both of which have soothing and anti-inflammatory properties on the skin.

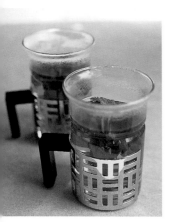

Fragrance oils may start out as essential oils, and often have similar names—Lavender Fragrance oil, for example—but they usually contain quantities of cheap synthetic versions of the chemicals found in essential oils. They should not be used on the skin, or for any health condition, since they are intended solely for use as "nice smells," and not for therapeutic applications. It is useful to compare the smells of the fragrance oils and essential oils, because you may find that your expectation of what an essential oil should smell like has been influenced by the many synthetic fragrances found in our society.

Herbal teas are another type of plant extract that contain small amounts of essential oils. Some of the essential oil in the herbs is

> **Caution:**
> Tinctures, infused oils, and fragrance oils should not be drunk or ingested. They must be kept out of the reach of children or anyone with impaired judgment.
> Always store essential oils in a cool dark place.

extracted when you pour boiling water onto them, but it will quickly evaporate if you don't cover the cup or teapot. The teas also contain water-soluble compounds, like the tinctures, and have different therapeutic properties from essential oils. The quantity of essential oil in a cup of herbal tea is much less than in one drop of oil.

Most people are familiar with vegetable oils, such as sunflower seed oil, olive oil, and sweet almond oil. These oils are made by the plants as a food source for the baby plant if the seeds should germinate. They have a greasy feel when you rub them between your fingers, they are not soluble in water, and they can be heated to high temperatures (e.g. 350°F/180°C) without evaporating. Vegetable oils are used therapeutically as dietary supplements, because they contain fat-soluble substances, such as Vitamin E. They are also used as emollients and skin nutrients by the cosmetics industry.

Below: Distillation equipment from the Renaissance. The woman is preparing the sample, while the man checks the furnace under the still.

Vegetable oils and diet

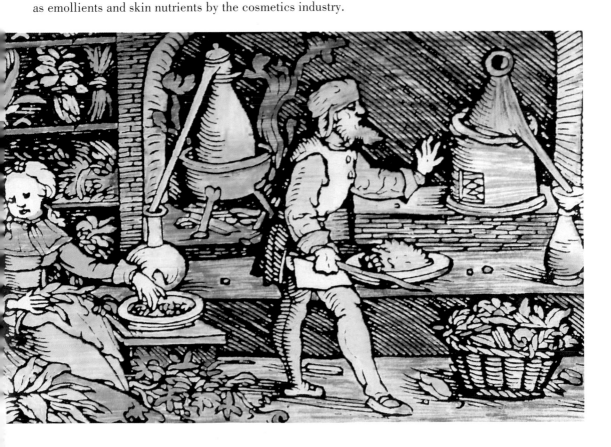

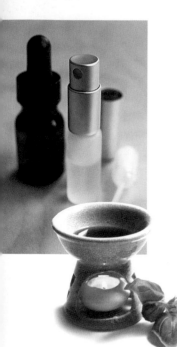

Above: Oils can be vaporized or, when diluted, used as a spritz.

Essential oils differ from vegetable oils in chemical structure, which is what gives them their characteristic aromas and therapeutic properties. Essential oils are nongreasy, and often feel slightly astringent or drying on the skin. This is because they dissolve the skin's natural oils and penetrate easily into the skin, whereas the vegetable oils largely remain on the surface. Essential oils are also fairly flammable, and evaporate most quickly at temperatures in the 104–180°F (40–80°C) range. Like vegetable oils, they do not dissolve in water. Essential oils have a range of therapeutic properties, including anti-inflammatory, antiseptic, relaxant, and wound-healing capabilities, but should not be used for cooking or flavoring food.

The branched and rigid chemical structures of essential oil molecules enable them to interact with specific olfactory receptors in our nasal cavity, which in turn means that we can smell them. The flexible, unbranched vegetable-oil molecules do not interact specifically with the olfactory receptors, and therefore have a faint smell compared with that of the essential oils.

Essential oils therefore carry the characteristic aroma of each plant. This is one of the reasons for naming them essences or essential oils. The odor produced by different herbs and flowers was thought to be the spiritual "signature," or perhaps even the soul, of the plant. This can make sense when you consider that an aroma is invisible, and yet it can immediately generate a mental image of what you are smelling. Even imagining the smell of a lemon (if you have smelled one before!) can bring to mind the image of the shiny yellow fruit. Like the vivid memory recall evoked by a smell, it seems almost magical.

Good vibrations

Some aromatherapists believe that essential oils carry a particular vibrational energy that can influence the energy fields of human beings. At present there are no scientifically valid tools for quantifying or predicting the effects of different oils in this regard. The oft-quoted Kirlian photography method that purports to photograph the aura or vibrational energy field of an object does not yield reproducible, scientifically meaningful results. This is not to say that the theory of vibrational energy is invalid, just that science has not yet measured it. Using essential oils from a vibrational perspective relies on the practitioner's intuition, experience, and sensitivity, and may overlap with faith healing and other forms of spiritual healing.

What can be measured with available scientific tools are the physiological effects that essential oils have on the body. The different three-dimensional

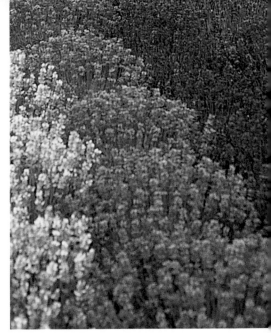

structures of the essential-oil molecules enable them to interact with structures in the human body, such as neurons, muscle cells, blood cells, and inflammatory proteins. This is an ongoing area of study, and new therapeutic effects of different plant molecules and their combinations are being discovered.

From a physiological point of view, the total chemical composition of an essential oil affects its therapeutic properties. If synthetic chemicals are added, this can significantly alter the natural balance of the oil's chemistry. Aromatherapists therefore prefer to use essential oils that are organic, harvested from wild plants, and extracted from a single source of plant material. Oils that satisfy these criteria are less likely to have had synthetics added.

It is important to bear in mind that essential oils are made up of a flexible combination of different compounds, varying within a range of percentages from year to year and batch to batch. Essential oils are like wines, and similar criteria influence their aroma and quality. For example, essential oils from the same botanic species—even propagated from the same plant—produce different combinations of chemicals when grown in different climatic conditions or geographical locations. An instance of this is *Lavandula angustifolia*, which produces a different aroma depending on whether it is grown at sea level or at high altitude.

Above: Fields of lavender are vulnerable to hybridization by pollinating insects. This can affect the chemical composition of the oil.

Left: The highest-quality oils are subject to a number of analytical tests, including chromatography (see over the page). This gas chromatograph chart of Tea Tree oil shows the percentage of each chemical constituent in the oil.

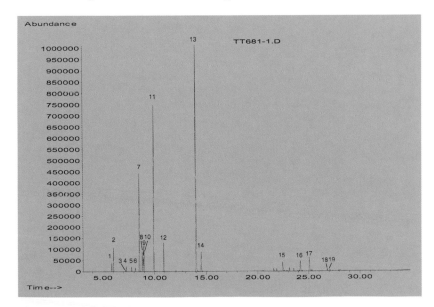

1 alpha-thujene	1.0
2 alpha-pinene	2.6
3 sabinene	0.2
4 beta-pinene	0.6
5 myrcene	0.6
6 alpha-phellandrene	0.4
7 alpha-terpinene	12.1
8 para-cymene	2.1
9 limonene+beta-phellandrene	1.8
10 1,8-cineole	2.5
11 gamma-terpinene	22.4
12 terpinolene	3.9
13 terpinen-4-ol	39.9
14 alpha-terpineol	2.9
15 aromadendrene	1.6
16 viridiflorene	2.1
17 delta-cadinene	2.3
18 globulol	0.3
19 viridiflorol	0.1
Total %	99.4

<table>
<tr><td>Quality control ❦</td><td>The essential oils from the same species that have a different chemical make-up are identified as different "chemotypes," see Rosemary (*Rosmarinus officinalis*), page 140. It has camphor and cineole chemotypes. However, most perfumers like their fragrance materials to smell the same year in and year out. This means that synthetic materials are often added to the essential oils to make them smell "right." This influences the quality of essential oils</td></tr>
</table>

available to aromatherapists. Until research demonstrates that synthetic materials do not affect the therapeutic properties of the oils, most aromatherapists prefer to avoid oils they know are altered. There is anecdotal evidence that the synthetic so-called "fragrance oils," which are available usually at much cheaper prices than essential oils, can cause headaches and skin irritation in ways that pure essential oils do not.

testing, testing

Specific gravity is the density of an oil compared with that of water. The density of essential oils is fairly consistent within a small range, so any additions may affect the density of an oil.

Optical rotation is the property of some essential oils to bend polarized light off a straight line by a certain number of degrees. Any additions that are optically active may alter the overall optical rotation of an oil.

Refractive index is the amount by which the oil deflects normal light from a straight path, in a similar way to a prism, and this also changes if the ratio of compounds alters.

Gas chromatography and mass spectroscopy machines identify types and percentages of chemicals in an essential oil. Together, the two machines can be used to determine the exact nature of each chemical.

Right: **1** Best-quality essential oils are subject to rigorous quality control.
2 Even the best machines are no substitute for the human nose! Organoleptic analysis (smelling) is the best test of whether you like an essential oil.

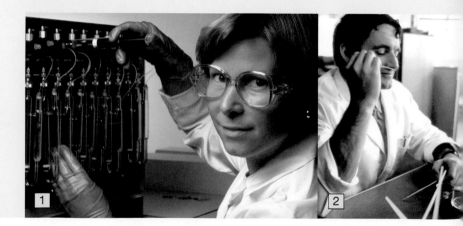

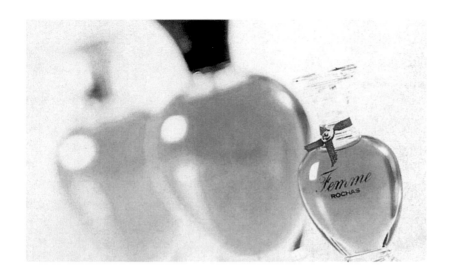

There are analytical techniques to assess the quality of essential oils, and most larger suppliers analyze each batch of oil to check that it meets their quality standards. Physical analyses, such as the determination of the specific gravity, optical rotation, or refractive index, allow for the comparison of a new oil with a standard sample.

Above: The most expensive perfume in the world, "Joy" by Jean Patou, contains precious extracts of rose and jasmine. Cheaper perfumes use synthetic fragrance compounds.

In spite of all the technological methods for analyzing essential oil quality, I suggest that enjoyment of the odor is the deciding factor in the purchase of an essential oil.

The human nose is a remarkably sensitive analytical instrument, capable in some cases of picking up substances in concentrations of parts per billion. For example, one of the key odorants in rose oil is beta-damascenone. It is present at a normal concentration of 0.14% in Rose oil, but because of the sensitivity of the human nose, which can detect it at 0.009 parts per billion in the air, it contributes nearly 70% of the oil's characteristic odor. So train your nose and enjoy exploring the fragrant world of essential oils.

The power of scent

The hedonic response to an odor is the extent to which a person likes or dislikes the odor. The offensiveness or pleasantness of an odor seems to have a strong effect on cognition and mood, with people reporting increased feelings of well-being and happiness in response to pleasant odors, and feelings of irritation, illness, tension, and inability to concentrate in response to unpleasant odors.

Hedonics: the benefits of pleasant aromas

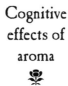

The hedonic response is used as a marker in the development of new food and fragrance products. There is also a branch of research dubbed "aromachology" (the psychology of aroma), which assesses the effects of odors on mood and cognitive function. Aromachologists examined the influence of food odors and other domestic aromas, and also studied the effects of essential-oil aromas. The overall conclusion was that smells people liked made them feel good, and smells they disliked made them feel bad—which concurs with common sense. Other studies have shown that odors perceived as unpleasant increased feelings of annoyance and made people more likely to report feeling sick. Laboratory tests showed that odors perceived as pleasant, on the other hand, seemed to promote people's feelings of relaxation, happiness, concentration, and alertness. Pleasant smells also improved mood and productivity in the workplace. One study showed that workers chose more efficient strategies and set higher goals for themselves in a pleasantly fragranced room than in a nonscented room.

Cognitive effects of aroma

The effects of odor on anxiety and claustrophobia have also been investigated. Magnetic Resonance Imaging (MRI) scanning, which requires people to lie still in a dark enclosed tube while images are taken of the functioning of their internal organs, causes claustrophobic anxiety in many people. Researchers found that heliotropin, a pleasant vanilla-like odor, appeared to be the most effective aroma in helping people manage their anxiety during MRI.

It is well known that odors can generate vivid recall of memories, especially memories with emotional content. Several of the essential oils, such as Rosemary, Peppermint, and Basil, have a reputation for stimulating memory processes and alertness, and a small amount of research has been carried out into these effects.

For example, one study showed that Rosemary oil vaporized in the air of the testing cubicle enhanced subjects' short- and longer-term memory, but that it slightly impaired the speed of memory recall compared with that of control subjects. In the same study, Lavender oil was associated with a significant decrease in memory performance, and slowed reaction times in memory and attention tasks, when compared with both Rosemary oil subjects and the control subjects.

Research from Japan confirmed that odors of some essential oils had a definite effect on brainwave patterns and cognitive function. Essential oils of Basil, Jasmine, Peppermint, Rose, and Ylang ylang all affected a brainwave pattern known as the Contingent Negative Variation in a way thought to indicate an increase in alertness; whereas German Chamomile, Lavender, and Sandalwood produced a different brainwave pattern, thought to indicate a decrease in alertness. Jasmine, Pine, Lemon, and Orange oils were all shown to reduce error rates in various clerical tasks— although the effect seemed to depend to a greater or lesser extent on odor liking. Some Japanese companies even add different oils to their air-conditioning units in order to improve their employees' productivity. Another area where pleasant aromas seem to be

having beneficial effects is in the management of difficult behaviors in people with dementia. Several studies suggest that the aroma of the oils helps reduce people's agitation and confusion. Pleasant aromas can also improve the environmental odor of residential care institutions, which in turn impacts on people's perception of how they are feeling.

Another human response to odor, known as odor conditioning, has potential usefulness in drug therapies. Odor conditioning is a protective mechanism. When people have experienced eating food that made them vomit, often smelling that food subsequently is enough to make them feel nauseous. The physical experience of vomiting is conditioned to the odor of the food. The principle of odor conditioning can be used to help people establish an aversion to a habit such as smoking.

Unfortunately, odors can be conditioned unintentionally during chemotherapy treatments for cancer or

| Odor conditioning ❧ |

AIDS. This can be a problem, since normally pleasant odors, such as those of nutritious food, can become triggers for nausea. This can lead to malnutrition and increased weakness, which obviously exacerbates the person's condition.

On the other hand, it is possible to link an odor with a drug that causes a beneficial physiological response, such as the immune response. In one case study investigating the treatment of lupus (chronic inflammatory disease characterized by fatigue, fever, and skin lesions), researchers paired chemotherapy drugs with Cod-liver oil and Rose essential oil for two dosages of the chemotherapy drugs. They found that the odor of Rose oil alone produced the desired immune response, and although they did not dare test how long the effect would last, they found they could administer the Rose oil in place of the drugs once in every two treatments. This increased the person's ability to tolerate the chemotherapy for longer.

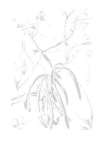

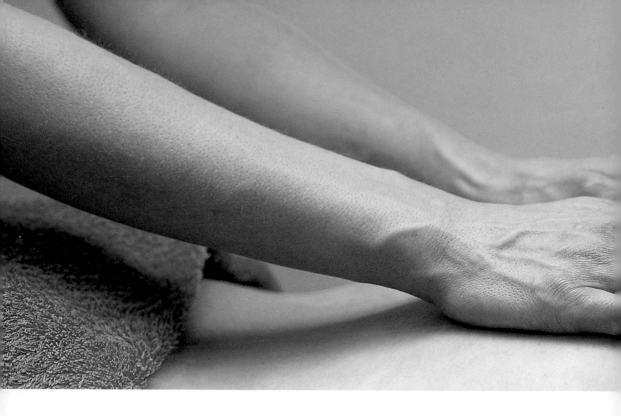

Massage and essential oils

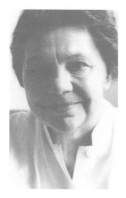

Above: Marguerite Maury
used aromatherapy in France,
as part of beauty therapy. In
the late 1950s, she
introduced it to England, from
where it spread to the rest of
the world.

In the previous section, the focus was on the use of essential oils for their influence on mood and cognition through the sense of smell. While this is how aromatherapy acquired its name, most aromatherapists are also trained in the practice of at least one type of massage. The essential oils are added to the massage oil and applied to the body. The combination of massage and the mood effects of the essential oils is a compelling aid to stress reduction.

There are many forms of massage, but essentially they are methods of touching with the intention to help. Massage can be either relaxing or stimulating, though it is most often associated with relaxation. Massage is effective in reducing stress and promoting the body's own natural healing responses. If a person is sick or stressed, the gentle nurturing touch of a massage can convey a sense of "safe space," which allows relaxation. The relaxation response to this sort of touch is evident even in babies.

Being in a state of relaxation allows the body to spend more of its energies on returning to balanced health instead of needing to maintain tight muscles and stiff postural patterns. Although it is obviously preferable to visit a

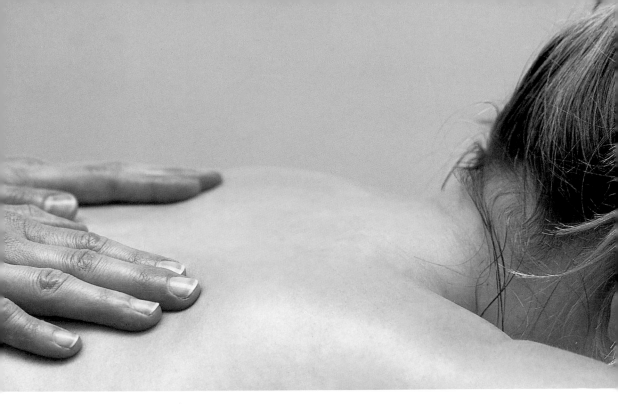

qualified massage therapist, there are techniques that you can do at home or at work to bring relief from stress and tension.

The following pages demonstrate some simple massage sequences for use in conjunction with essential oil blends, to be vaporized, or applied directly to the skin during the massage. You can do them on yourself, or on another person, or have someone do them for you. The essential oil blends are recommendations only, and as you become familiar with the oils, you will be able to experiment with your own blends. It would also be helpful to ask a qualified aromatherapist to make up a blend for you, which you can then use for your own massages.

Key points to remember

If you are pregnant, breastfeeding, or have an existing health condition such as epilepsy, consult a health practitioner about the appropriateness of any massage technique.

• Arrange the space so that you will not be interrupted.

• Communicate nurture, gentleness, and love in your touch.

• If it hurts, stop.

• Do not apply essential oils to the skin of babies under 24 months old, to anyone unable to communicate, to broken skin, rashes, or burns.

• Avoid mucous membranes and eyes.

• Wash your hands afterward and put the sheets and clothes in the laundry.

Temples and scalp: stress relief

Stress relief vaporizer blend:

1 drop each of Mandarin, Lavender, and Frankincense oils.

Temples and scalp hold considerable amounts of tension. This massage can be done with or without oils, at home or at work. If you do use oil, pour a small amount of vegetable oil into your hands, so that they are only slightly greasy when you rub them together. Add 1 drop of Lavender oil, if desired.

1 Using your fingertips, gently push the skin in small circles over the temple bones. This stretches and releases the fine muscles around the eyes and ears. It is easier to get someone to do this for you.

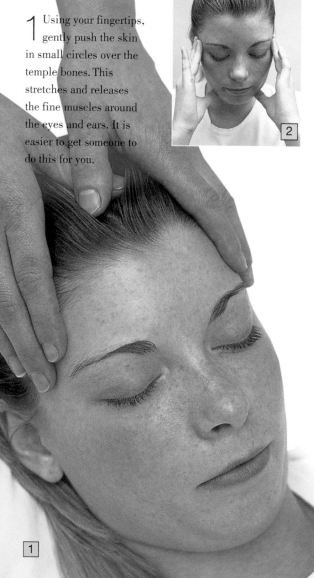

1

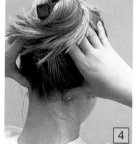

2

2 Using both hands, one on either side of the face, drag the tips of the middle three fingers down the jawline from the temples. Brace with thumbs under the jaw.

3

3 Using thumb and forefinger, squeeze the eyebrows, starting at the nose, moving out toward the temples.

4

4 Place the fingertips and thumb of each hand on either side of the head behind the ears. As in step 1, aim to move the skin in small circles across the bones of the scalp. Massage the entire scalp.

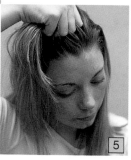

5

5 Grasp handfuls of hair near the roots, and tighten your grasp, pulling gently on the roots. Move the handfuls until the whole scalp has been pulled.

Face: relaxation

Relaxing face massage blend:
1 teaspoon of Sweet Almond oil, with 1 drop of either Neroli, Rose, Sandalwood, Jasmine, or Frankincense oils.

A face massage can be intimate and deeply relaxing. Set the scene with quiet music and low light levels. The person receiving the massage should lie comfortably on his or her back, with the head supported by a cushion. Use as little vegetable oil as possible, so that the skin does not feel greasy.

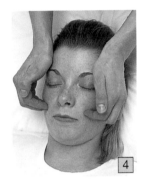

4 Resting the balls of the hands on the eyebrows, cradle the cheeks in your fingers. If you want to do a longer massage, add the Temple and Scalp massage moves after step 1.

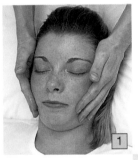

1 Apply the oil to the entire face with your fingertips, going from the center line out to the sides, starting at the hairline and moving down to the chin.

2 Using the tips of your forefingers, trace arches following the eyebrows from the center to the sides of the forehead, moving from eyebrows to hairline.

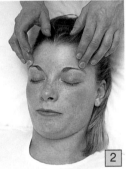

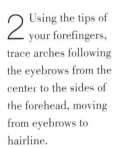

3 Trace a circle around the eyes with your forefingers: Between the eyebrows, across the eyebrows, and back up the side of the nose.

5 Press gently on the skin on either side of the nostrils, and hold for 5–10 seconds. Release and repeat. This can also help with sinus pain.

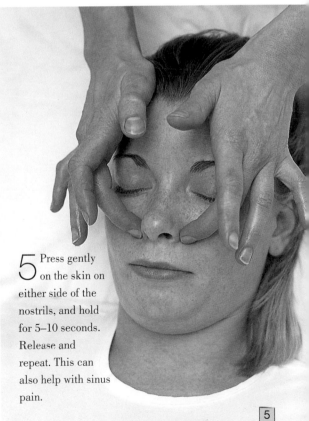

Neck and shoulders:
tension relief

Vaporizer focus blend:

1 drop each of Lemon, Rosemary (cineole chemotype), and Basil (methyl chavicol chemotype) oils.

Tension relief massage blend:

1 teaspoon of vegetable oil with 1 drop of Lavender oil, and 5 drops of prediluted (3%) German Chamomile oil.

Caution:
When using hot tap water, always check that it is not too hot.

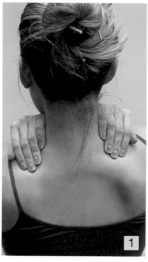
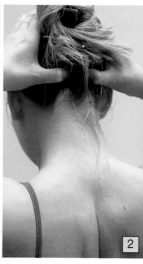
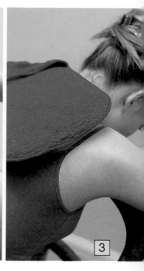

1 Use fingers and palm to squeeze the shoulder muscles at the bottom of the neck, and work outward to the shoulder with several squeezing movements. Do both sides.

2 Take the back of the head in both hands, and using your thumbs gently press up into the soft area underneath the skull at the top of the neck. Start at the center and work around to the ears.

3 Warm a heat pack according to the manufacturer's instructions, and place it across the shoulders and back of the neck for 5–10 minutes. Or make a warm compress with a towel and warm water to use in the same way.

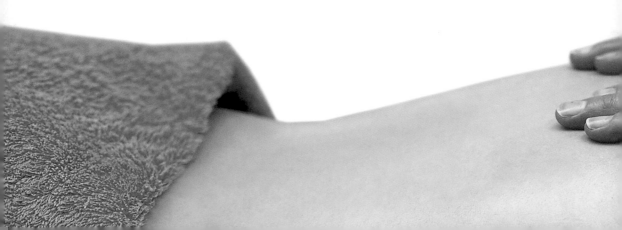

The neck and shoulders also hold stress, and tension there can cause headaches and a lack of focus or concentration. These techniques can be done without undressing. If using oil, the tension relief blend will help ease tension and stress.

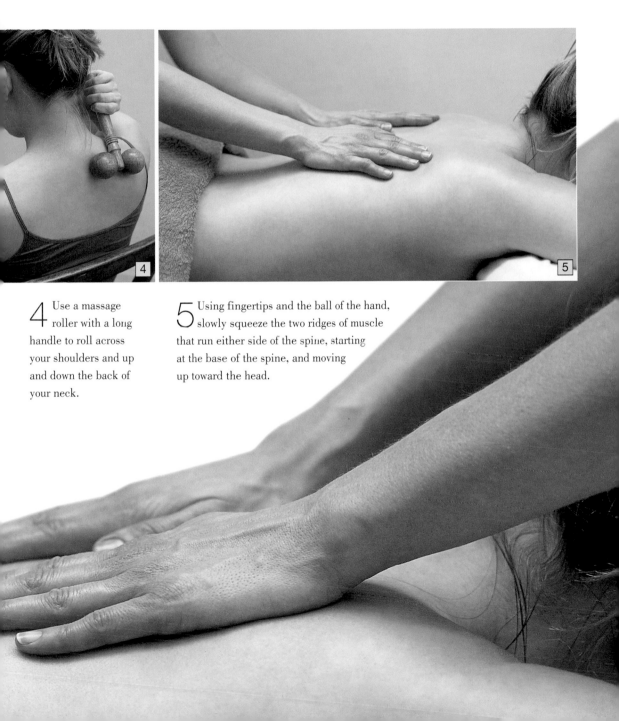

4 Use a massage roller with a long handle to roll across your shoulders and up and down the back of your neck.

5 Using fingertips and the ball of the hand, slowly squeeze the two ridges of muscle that run either side of the spine, starting at the base of the spine, and moving up toward the head.

Back: relaxation

Massage blend:
1 tablespoon of vegetable oil, and 2 drops each of Lavender and Sandalwood oil. Add 1 drop of Ylang ylang oil for sensuality.

Back massage needs some preparation if it is done unclothed, and with oil. Use a massage table, or arrange a floor space or bed with old towels and pillows, in case of staining, to make it comfortable for the person to lie face down, preferably without twisting the neck to one side. Cover the other parts of the body in towels or a blanket. If the massage is done clothed, do the moves with the person sitting facing backward on a chair.

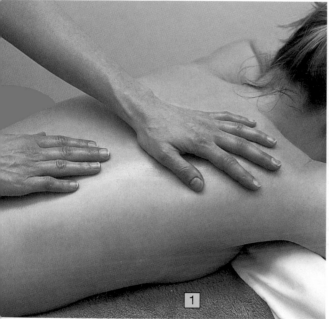

1

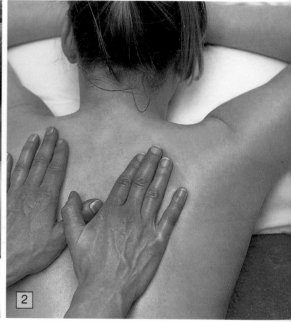

2

1 Using palms and fingers, apply the oil blend to the body in short strokes from base of spine to shoulders. Use more vegetable oil, if required.

2 Slide palms up the back, close to either side of the spine, from base to neck, and come back down the sides. Repeat in a circular, flowing motion.

3 Keeping the palm in contact with the skin, gently knead the muscles all over the back, paying attention to the shoulder area.

4 Keeping your fingers on the person's shoulders, move your thumbs up across the shoulder muscles in firm circular strokes. Also use the Neck and Shoulders techniques, as shown on the previous page.

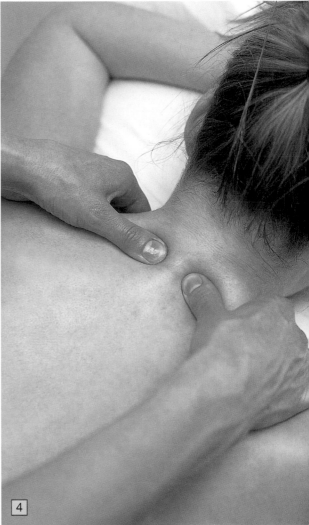

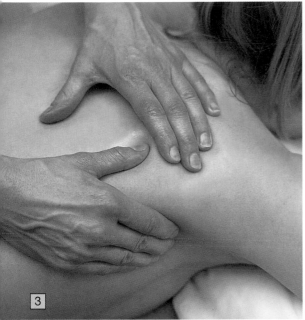

3

4

5 Run your thumbs in small firm strokes up the ridges of muscle on either side of the spine. Finish by repeating step 2 several times.

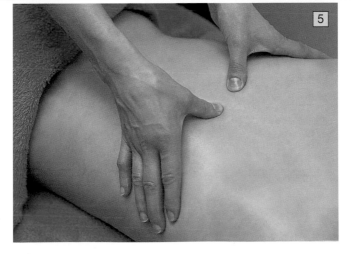

5

Hands: nurture

Nurturing vaporizer blend:
2 drops of Vanilla, 1 drop of Mandarin oil—or use a favorite oil.

Stiff joints massage blend:
1 teaspoon of vegetable oil with 1 drop each of Black Pepper, Rosemary (either chemotype), and German Chamomile oil. Alternatively, use a hand cream. Do steps 1 to 5 on one hand at a time.

When a person is confined to bed, a hand massage can be very soothing and nurturing. Hand massage can also be helpful for people with stiff joints in the hands, because massage stimulates blood circulation—though care must be taken if the joints are swollen and tender.

1 Holding the person's hand, gently slide your thumbs up each gap between the finger bones on the back of the hand, from the base of the fingers to the wrists.

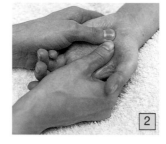

2

3 Support the person's hand and use the thumb and fingers of your other hand to gently twist and knead each joint, starting at the base of each finger.

2 Turn the hand over, and make small circles with your thumbs over the palm, moving the flesh over the muscles and bones. Pay attention to the base of the thumb.

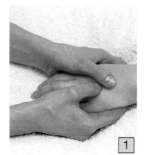

1

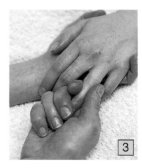

3

4 Take the hand in both your hands, as in step 1, and gently squeeze it, moving the bones in the hand and gently moving the wrist, as you hold the hand.

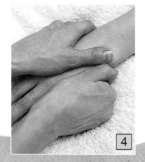

4

5 Sandwich the hand between your palms, and maintain a constant gentle pressure for several seconds. Slowly release the pressure and place the person's hand down.

5

Feet: easing the ache

Tired, aching feet respond well to foot baths and massage. If the feet are too ticklish at first, wrap them in a towel and massage through the towel. Do not massage if there are infections, such as athlete's foot (tinea), because this can spread the infection. Make sure that the knee and leg are supported during the massage, and massage one foot at a time.

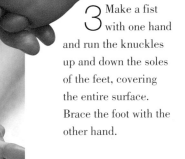

3

Refreshing foot bath blend:
Add 2 drops of Lavender oil and 1 drop of Peppermint oil to a foot bath or bowl of warm water large enough to put two feet in comfortably.

1 Soak feet in a warm foot bath, or soak a towel in hot water and wrap it around the feet like a compress. Dry gently with a towel.

3 Make a fist with one hand and run the knuckles up and down the soles of the feet, covering the entire surface. Brace the foot with the other hand.

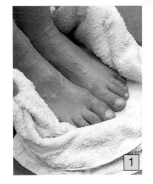

2

Anti-infection foot bath blend:
Add 3 drops of Tea Tree and 1 drop of Lemongrass oil to a foot bath of warm water.

2 Apply the oil and squeeze the foot all over with both hands, thumbs on the sole. The aim is to move the bones in the feet gently around.

Foot massage blend:
2 teaspoons of vegetable oil, 3 drops of Bergamot oil, 2 drops of Virginian Cedarwood oil.

1

5

5 Holding each foot in turn in your hands, use your thumbs to press firmly all over the sole. Include the toes if not too ticklish.

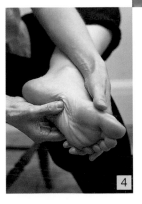

4 Massage the inner side of the foot with your thumb, from toe to heel, supporting the foot with the other hand. This area can be tender, so proceed gently.

4

Therapeutic properties of
Essential Oils

Body Part	Ailment	Oils	Body Part	Ailment	Oils
Skin	Acne	Matricaria chamomilla, Citrus aurantium (Petitgrain), Citrus latifolia, Melaleuca alternifolia	Nails	Infected nails	Cymbopogon winterianus, Cymbopogon citratus, Melaleuca alternifolia
	Boils	Cymbopogon winterianus, Melaleuca alternifolia, Thymus vulgaris	Muscles	Aches and pains, stiffness	
	Bruises	Helichrysum italicum		and strain	Laurus nobilis, Melaleuca
	Burns	Lavandula angustifolia			leucadendron, Lavandula latifolia,
	Cellulite	Cupressus sempervirens, Citrus paradisii, Citrus sinensis			Melaleuca quinquinervia, Myristica fragrans, Myrtus communis, Pinus
	Cold sores	Melissa officinalis			pinaster, Rosmarinus officinalis,
	Dermatitis	Matricaria chamomilla, Santalum album, Vetivera zizanoides			Vetivera zizanoides
	Dryness	Aniba rosaeodora, Boswellia carterii, Cymbopogon martinii, Rosa damascena, Santalum album		Sprains	Helichrysum italicum, Lavandula latifolia
	Eczema	Styrax benzoin, Matricaria chamomilla, Pogostemon cablin, Vetivera zizanoides	Joints	Arthritis	Laurus nobilis, Melaleuca leucadendron, Zingiber officinale, Lavandula latifolia,
	Edema	Cupressus sempervirens, Citrus paradisii			Melaleuca quinquinervia, Thymus vulgaris,
	Facial redness	Matricaria chamomilla, Rosa damascena			Vetivera zizanoides
	Fungal infections	Cymbopogon citratus, Melaleuca alternifolia		Rheumatism	Melaleuca quinquinervia, Vetivera zizanoides
	Grazes and cuts	Origanum majorana, Commiphora myrrha		Swollen joints	Juniperus communis, Lavandula latifolia, Vetivera zizanoides
	Insect bites and stings	Matricaria chamomilla, Lavandula angustifolia	Circulation	High blood pressure	Origanum majorana
	Oily skin	Pelargonium graveolens, Juniperus communis, Citrus aurantium (Petitgrain)		Poor circulation, cold hands and feet	Piper nigrum, Cardamomum elettaria, Rosmarinus officinalis, Thymus vulgaris
	Pimples	Thymus vulgaris			
	Psoriasis	Styrax benzoin, Pogostemon cablin			
	Shaving rash	Citrus latifolia, Melaleuca alternifolia	Head	Headaches	Lavandula angustifolia, Mentha piperita
	Shingles	Pelargonium graveolens			
	Skin ulcers	Achillea millefolium			
	Tinea (athlete's foot)	Cymbopogon citratus, Melaleuca alternifolia	Eyes	Blephoritis	Matricaria chamomilla
				Itchy eyes	Matricaria chamomilla
	Unpleasant body odor	Cymbopogon martinii	Stomach	Nausea	Zingiber officinale, Mentha spicata
	Warts	Citrus limonum		Poor appetite	Laurus nobilis, Citrus sinensis, Vanilla planifolia
	Wounds	Achillea millefolium, Canarium luzonicum, Commiphora myrrha		Travel sickness	Mentha spicata
	Wrinkles	Aniba rosaeodora, Boswellia carterii, Commiphora myrrha, Cymbopogon martinii	Intestines	Colic	Zingiber officinale, Mentha spicata
				Constipation	Pimpinella anisum
				Cramps	Achillea millefolium, Mentha piperita
				Flatulence	Pimpinella anisum, Cardamomum elettaria
				Hemorrhoids	Cupressus sempervirens

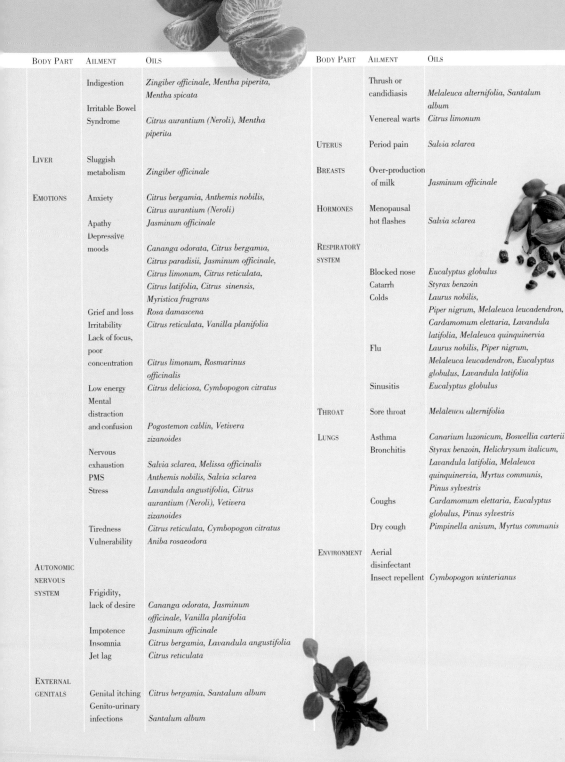

Body Part	Ailment	Oils
	Indigestion	Zingiber officinale, Mentha piperita, Mentha spicata
	Irritable Bowel Syndrome	Citrus aurantium (Neroli), Mentha piperita
LIVER	Sluggish metabolism	Zingiber officinale
EMOTIONS	Anxiety	Citrus bergamia, Anthemis nobilis, Citrus aurantium (Neroli)
	Apathy	Jasminum officinale
	Depressive moods	Cananga odorata, Citrus bergamia, Citrus paradisii, Jasminum officinale, Citrus limonum, Citrus reticulata, Citrus latifolia, Citrus sinensis, Myristica fragrans
	Grief and loss	Rosa damascena
	Irritability	Citrus reticulata, Vanilla planifolia
	Lack of focus, poor concentration	Citrus limonum, Rosmarinus officinalis
	Low energy	Citrus deliciosa, Cymbopogon citratus
	Mental distraction and confusion	Pogostemon cablin, Vetivera zizanoides
	Nervous exhaustion	Salvia sclarea, Melissa officinalis
	PMS	Anthemis nobilis, Salvia sclarea
	Stress	Lavandula angustifolia, Citrus aurantium (Neroli), Vetivera zizanoides
	Tiredness	Citrus reticulata, Cymbopogon citratus
	Vulnerability	Aniba rosaeodora
AUTONOMIC NERVOUS SYSTEM	Frigidity, lack of desire	Cananga odorata, Jasminum officinale, Vanilla planifolia
	Impotence	Jasminum officinale
	Insomnia	Citrus bergamia, Lavandula angustifolia
	Jet lag	Citrus reticulata
EXTERNAL GENITALS	Genital itching	Citrus bergamia, Santalum album
	Genito-urinary infections	Santalum album

Body Part	Ailment	Oils
	Thrush or candidiasis	Melaleuca alternifolia, Santalum album
	Venereal warts	Citrus limonum
UTERUS	Period pain	Salvia sclarea
BREASTS	Over-production of milk	Jasminum officinale
HORMONES	Menopausal hot flashes	Salvia sclarea
RESPIRATORY SYSTEM		
	Blocked nose	Eucalyptus globulus
	Catarrh	Styrax benzoin
	Colds	Laurus nobilis, Piper nigrum, Melaleuca leucadendron, Cardamomum elettaria, Lavandula latifolia, Melaleuca quinquinervia
	Flu	Laurus nobilis, Piper nigrum, Melaleuca leucadendron, Eucalyptus globulus, Lavandula latifolia
	Sinusitis	Eucalyptus globulus
THROAT	Sore throat	Melaleuca alternifolia
LUNGS	Asthma Bronchitis	Canarium luzonicum, Boswellia carterii, Styrax benzoin, Helichrysum italicum, Lavandula latifolia, Melaleuca quinquinervia, Myrtus communis, Pinus sylvestris
	Coughs	Cardamomum elettaria, Eucalyptus globulus, Pinus sylvestris
	Dry cough	Pimpinella anisum, Myrtus communis
ENVIRONMENT	Aerial disinfectant	
	Insect repellent	Cymbopogon winterianus

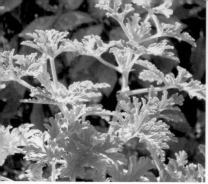
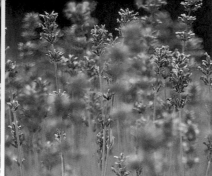
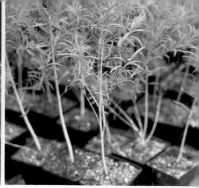

Skin

Some essential oils can help to alleviate pain and inflammation, and promote rapid healing of the skin.

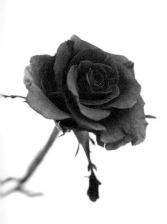

Allergic responses:

When using oils directly on the skin, always do a patch test first.

If you experience any irritation, wipe off with vegetable oil and flush the area with cold running water. See Safety Tips, page 9.

OILS

Oils often used for skin ailments are:

Lavandula angustifolia (Lavender): Anti-inflammatory, antiseptic, and skin-regenerative properties.

Matricaria chamomilla (German Chamomile): Excellent for reducing pain and inflammation.

Melaleuca alternifolia (Tea Tree): Prevention and cure of bacterial infection.

Commiphora myrrha (Myrrh): Anti-inflammatory, promotes skin repair.

AILMENTS

Insect bites, stings, small burns, cuts, abrasions need immediate treatment. The oils can be applied directly to the skin without diluting in vegetable oil—unless you happen to be allergic to them, in which case try *Santalum album* (Sandalwood).

Itchy dry skin can respond well to the anti-inflammatory oils mentioned above, though consult with your dermatologist if you have eczema, dermatitis, or psoriasis.

Acne, pimples often respond well to diluted *Pelargonium graveolens* (Geranium) and *Rosa damascena* (Rose):

5 drops in 1 teaspoon of Jojoba oil or Vitamin E cream.

Cellulite, sluggish circulation can be helped by oils that have diuretic properties or that stimulate the circulation, such as *Citrus paradisii* (Grapefruit), *Juniperus communis* (Juniper), and *Cupressus sempervirens* (Cypress). With chronic imbalances like these, use the oils in dilution (2 drops of each in 1 teaspoon of vegetable oil).

> Caution: If a cut or burn is larger than ¼–¾ in. (1–2 cm) long, seek medical advice, rather than treating the condition yourself.

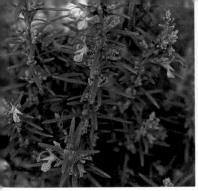 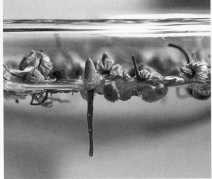 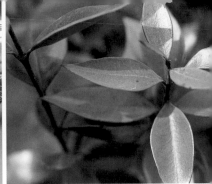

Muscles

There are some essential oils that are especially effective in alleviating muscle pain and inflammation.

OILS

Oils often used for muscle ailments are:

Rosmarinus officinalis (Rosemary): Increases bloodflow to muscles, creates warmth.

Myrtus communis (Myrtle): Increases bloodflow, has a mild painkilling effect.

Lavandula angustifolia (Lavender): anti-inflammatory.

Mentha piperita (Peppermint): Temporary numbing and painkilling effects; increases dermal bloodflow.

Thymus vulgaris (Thyme) CT linalool: Increases bloodflow to muscles; creates warmth.

AILMENTS

Joint diseases, **rheumatism** also cause muscular pain, but require different approaches. In osteoarthritis, it is mainly the larger skeletal joints that are affected, and the surrounding muscles often stiffen as a protection against the pain in the joint. The essential oils mentioned above that are warming and increase local bloodflow would be helpful here. In rheumatoid arthritis, however, it is the smaller joints, such as those in the hands, that are affected, and the main principle in the disease is inflammation of the synovial membrane around the joints. In this case, it is more helpful to use anti-inflammatory oils, such as *Lavandula angustifolia* (Lavender) and *Matricaria chamomilla* (German Chamomile).

> Caution:
> Thyme oil should be tested on the skin before use over a large area (5 drops to 1 teaspoon of vegetable oil). Do not use if irritation results.
>   All Mint oils should be used with care as they can inflame mucous membranes.

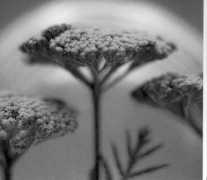
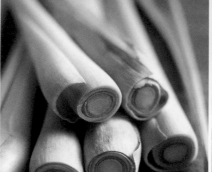
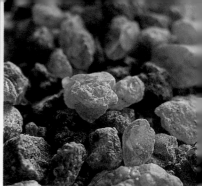

Germs and infections

Many essential oils have antibacterial and antifungal properties, and help to dry up excess mucous and soothe inflammation caused by an infection.

OILS

Oils recommended for use in respiratory tract infections are:

Melaleuca alternifolia (Tea Tree): Anti-infectious, immune stimulant.

Achillea millefolium (Yarrow): Anti-inflammatory, mucolytic, expectorant, anti-infectious.

Melaleuca leucadendron (Cajuput): Mucolytic, expectorant.

Myrtus communis (Myrtle): Anti-infectious, mucolytic.

AILMENTS

Colds, influenza, coughs, sore throats are best treated by the inhalation method of each oil listed. Add 2 drops of essential oil to a bowl of hot tap water, and inhale the vapors for up to 15 minutes, 3–4 times a day.

Painful coughs require soothing inhalation oils, such as *Styrax benzoin* (Benzoin) and *Santalum album* (Sandalwood). They can be diluted 5 drops to 1 teaspoon of vegetable oil for rubbing onto the throat and chest.

Candidiasis (thrush), the fungal infection, can

be treated with *Melaleuca alternifolia* (Tea Tree).

Inflammation, itching can be soothed with *Lavandula angustifolia* (Lavender) or *Santalum album* (Sandalwood).

Athlete's foot (tinea), a common fungal infection of the feet, can be treated with *Melaleuca alternifolia* (Tea Tree) and *Cymbopogon citratus* (Lemongrass). Use a blend of 1 drop of each oil (or 5 drops of one oil) in 1 teaspoon of vegetable oil, and apply to the affected area 3–4 times a day.

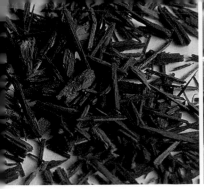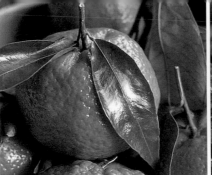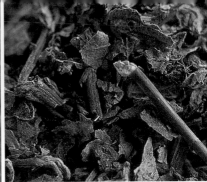

Stress

Of all the conditions that cause an imbalance in the healthy functioning of our bodies, stress is one of the most pervasive, and one of the most difficult to treat. There are often many interrelated causes of stress, which call for a holistic management approach. Although essential oils and aromatherapy can help you to manage stress, it is important to try and modify external and internal causes, wherever possible.

Essential oils can help with the following stress-related problems:

AILMENTS

Sleep disturbances

Vaporize 3 drops of either of these oils, or add the same quantity to a warm bath, before going to sleep:

Lavandula angustifolia (Lavender): Sedative, relaxant.

Anthemis nobilis (Roman Chamomile): Reduces anxiety, sedative.

Lack of concentration

Vaporize 2 drops of each of these oils together:

Citrus limonum (Lemon): Increases concentration, lifts mood.

Rosmarinus officinalis CT cineole (Rosemary): Increases focus and enhances some aspects of memory.

Feelings of helplessness, depression

Vaporize 3 drops of a combination of any of the following:

Citrus bergamia (Bergamot): Uplifting, relaxing, euphoric.

Citrus aurantium (Neroli): Uplifting, euphoric.

Citrus deliciosa (Mandarin): Uplifting, joyous.

Cananga odorata (Ylang ylang): Euphoric.

Emotional instability

Take a warm bath with 3 drops of any, or a combination, of the following:

Pogostemon cablin (Patchouli): Emotionally stabilizing, grounding.

Vetivera zizanoides (Vetiver): Relaxing, calming.

Santalum album (Sandalwood): Grounding, relaxing.

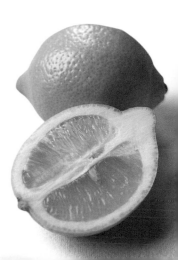

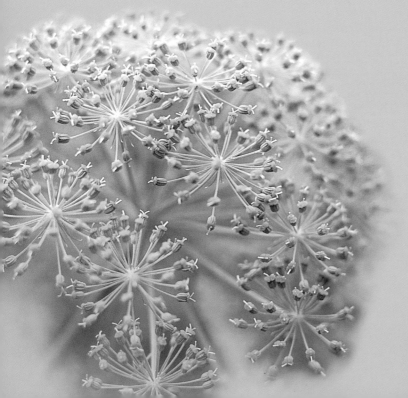

SECTION 2

the directory
of essential oils

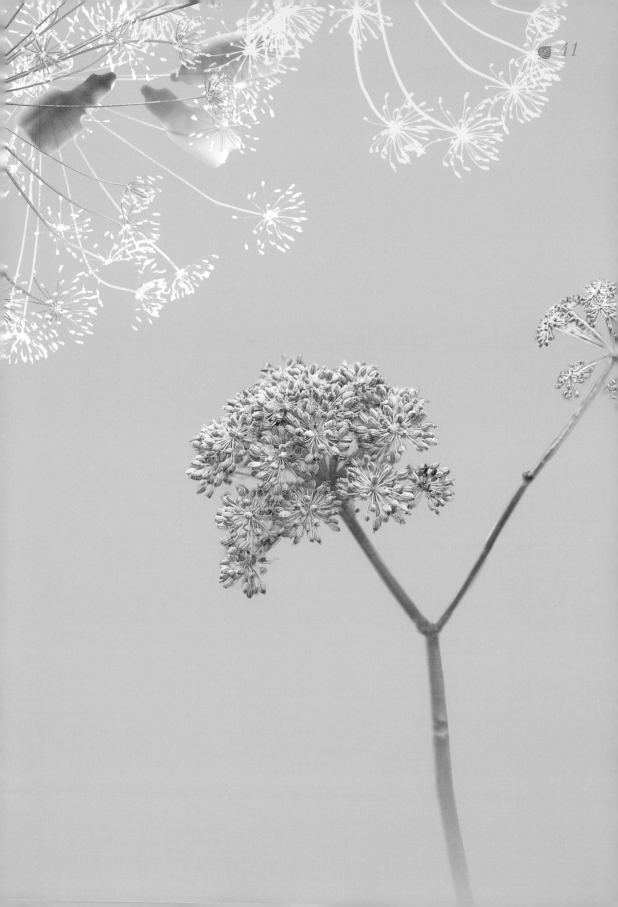

Abies alba

Fir, White

Many different species of Fir tree produce essential oils.
White Fir (*Abies alba*) is the sweetest and softest of the
Fir oils and is used in aromatherapy for this reason.
Douglas Fir (*Pseudotsuga menziesii*) and Balsamic Fir
(*A. balsamea*) yield essential oils with a more woody,
balsamic odor. The Balsamic Fir—also known as
Canadian Fir or Canadian Turpentine—is often used
as a Christmas tree because of its lovely shape.

The aerial parts of Fir trees are all aromatic. The essential oil used in aromatherapy is extracted from the needles by steam distillation and is sometimes known as Fir Needle oil for this reason. Perfume makers often add it to men's fragrances, or products designed to conjure images of the wild fresh outdoors.

Traditional aromatherapy uses

White Fir oil is used as a milder substitute for Pine oil (*Pinus pinaster*, see page 132) to treat stiff and sore muscles, or coughs with a lot of mucous. It is also used to stimulate bloodflow where there is poor circulation.

Ailments and remedies

Respiratory infections Put 1–2 drops of White Fir oil into a bowl of hot tap water, and inhale the vapors, covering your head with a towel to keep the vapors contained.

Muscular aches and pains Add 5 drops of White Fir oil to 1 tablespoon of vegetable oil, and massage into the affected area as required.

Why it works

The chemical constituents of White Fir oil do not seem to support its use in aromatherapy, but this may be due to variations between batches.

Limonene has antitumorigenic and bile-stimulant properties, although White Fir oil has not been used for this purpose in aromatherapy.

Alpha-pinene has mild antiseptic and warming properties, and probably contributes to the expectorant effect. It is likely that the percentage of alpha-pinene in the oil varies from season to season, and from one oil to

Fir, White

Active constituents

limonene **54.5%**
alpha-pinene **7.4%**
beta-caryophyllene **2.3%**

Other known constituents

camphene **14%**
santene **5%**
borneol **1%**
bornyl acetate **1%**

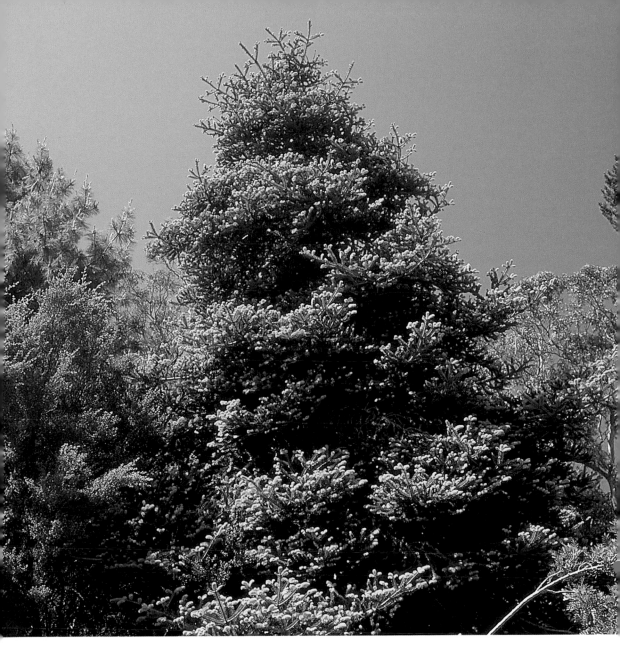

another. Industrial analyses of oils often exclude minor components, which may be the more active ingredients.

Beta-caryophyllene would contribute some anti-inflammatory properties, though at such small percentages, it is unlikely to be the major source of these.

Caution: The limonene in the oil can oxidize to form compounds that cause skin sensitization. Keep the bottle tightly sealed in a cool, dark place to minimize the oxidation process. Do not use White Fir oil on the skin if stored for more than one year.

Achillea millefolium

Yarrow

Yarrow is a herb from the Umbelliferae family, like Sweet Fennel, and grows wild along the roadside and in fields over most of Europe and North America. Its white or yellow flowerheads are distinctive in summer, and the entire plant exudes a pungent herbaceous aroma. Yarrow oil is aromatically similar to Clary Sage oil (see page 142), although the odor varies according to where and when the Yarrow was harvested. The oil can range in color from dark blue to pale yellow depending on the country of origin.

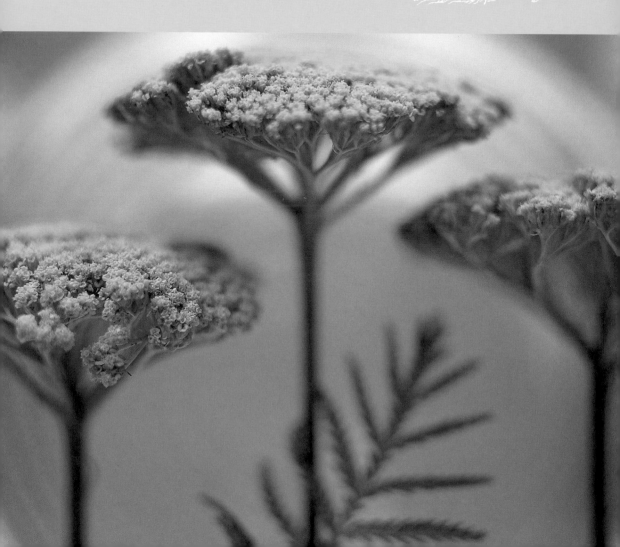

There is a long herbal tradition of using a Yarrow infusion as a wound-healing agent, and it was also thought to stop bleeding, especially from battle wounds. A tea made of Yarrow leaves is supposed to cause sweating, and thereby break the fever in colds and influenza. However, these effects are unlikely to be due to the essential oil.

Traditional aromatherapy uses

Yarrow oil is used for the treatment of cuts and abrasions because of its anti-inflammatory and antibacterial properties. Some sources suggest it may be useful for menstrual difficulties, such as regulating menstrual cycles or relieving menstrual pain. It may also be useful in the treatment of hemorrhoids, but be sure to consult your doctor first.

Ailments and remedies

Cuts and abrasions Add 5 drops of blue Yarrow oil to a bowl of warm water, and gently bathe the cut or abrasion in the water.

Cramps Add 5 drops of Yarrow oil to 1 tablespoon of vegetable oil and massage onto the affected area. If the cramps are abdominal, massage the abdomen in a clockwise direction, starting at the bottom of the belly on the person's right side. Massaging the lower back can also be helpful for abdominal cramps.

Why it works

Camphor has been shown to have relaxant effects on capillary smooth muscles, causing a rush of blood to an area. This makes Yarrow oil useful in sports liniments (see Caution).

1,8-Cineole is thought to be an expectorant, and has been used in chest rub preparations for the treatment of bronchitis, colds, and influenza. It also has mild anti-inflammatory properties on the respiratory linings.

Iso-artemisia ketone has possible antimalarial properties (see Caution).

Azulenes are thought to contribute anti-inflammatory properties. It is the azulene content that makes the oil blue: the deeper the shade of blue, the more azulenes it contains.

Achilline is a lactone compound that may cause allergic reactions.

Yarrow

Active constituents

camphor **17.7%**
1,8-cineole **9.5%**
iso-artemisia ketone **8.6%**
azulenes (variable)
achilline (variable)

Other significant constituents

sabinene **12.3%**
alpha-pinene **9.4%**
beta-pinene **7.3%**
terpinen-4-ol **4.3%**
borneol **2.5%**
thujone (variable).

Caution:
Yarrow oil is not recommended for internal use as camphor, thujone, and iso-artemisia ketone may have neurotoxic properties. Yarrow oil is contraindicated during pregnancy and for epileptics because of its possible neurotoxicity.

Angelica archangelica

Angelica

Angelica is a herb from the Umbelliferae family, which is most widely cultivated in Europe. In herbal tradition, the root was considered a cure-all. Its name may derive from the fact that it bloomed on the Christian holy day of the Archangel Michael. The hollow stems are cultivated for use as candied confectionery, and the stems and seeds flavor French liqueurs, such as Chartreuse.

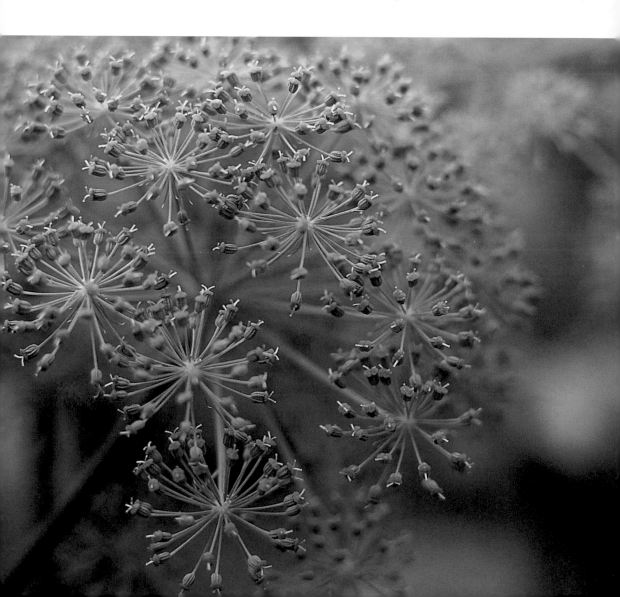

A pale yellow essential oil is extracted by steam distillation from the powdered dried root. Compounds in the root oil are thought to exercise a beneficial effect on women's hormones, and also to stimulate the immune system. An oil can be extracted from the seeds, which is possibly more suitable for the treatment of indigestion than the root oil.

Traditional aromatherapy uses

Angelica Root oil is most often used for premenstrual syndrome and painful periods. It is also used as an expectorant, and is thought to be helpful in stimulating the immune system.

Ailments and remedies

Premenstrual syndrome (PMS) Use 1 drop of Angelica Root oil on a tissue, tucked into the bra strap, to allow the odor of the oil to rise during the day. Or add 3 drops of Angelica Root oil to 1 tablespoon of vegetable oil and massage the abdomen in gentle clockwise circles, starting at the person's bottom right-hand side. You can also massage the lower back with this blend, but do not go out into the sun in a bikini afterward (see Caution).

Respiratory infections Put 1–2 drops of Angelica Root oil into a bowl of hot tap water, and inhale the vapors, covering your head with a towel to keep the vapors contained.

Why it works

Alpha-pinene has mild antiseptic and warming properties, and probably contributes to the expectorant effect.

1,8-cineole is a good expectorant, but is not present in all Angelica oils. If the oil has a eucalyptus odor, 1,8-cineole will be present in high enough quantities to indicate expectorant effects.

Ambrettolide, pentadecanolide, and the other musk compounds give the oil its earthy, musky odor, and may also be responsible when inhaled for its reputed effect on female hormones.

Angelica

Active constituents

alpha-pinene **25%**
1,8-cineole **14.5%**
ambrettolide **0.3%**
pentadecanolide **0.2%**

Other known constituents

alpha-phellandrene **13.5%**
limonene **8%**
borneol **1%**
bornyl acetate **<1%**
umbelliferone **<1%**
angelicine **<1%**
bergaptene **<1%**

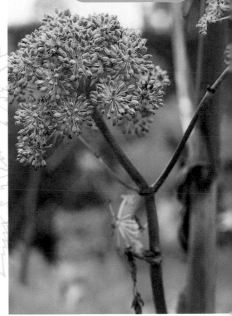

Caution: Do not go out into the sun or use a UV-ray lamp for 12 hours after application of Angelica Root oil to the skin. It can cause photosensitization due to the bergaptene content.

Aniba rosaeodora

Rosewood {or Bois-de-Rose}

Rosewood oil is extracted by steam distillation of wood chips from the heartwood of an Amazonian rainforest tree. The oil has been used extensively in perfumery and cosmetics for its lovely, soft, flowery scent. A similar oil is produced by the leaves of the Chinese Ho plant *Cinnamomum camphora* (linalool chemotype). The leaves of *Aniba rosaeodora* also produce an essential oil, which is less valued but smells similar.

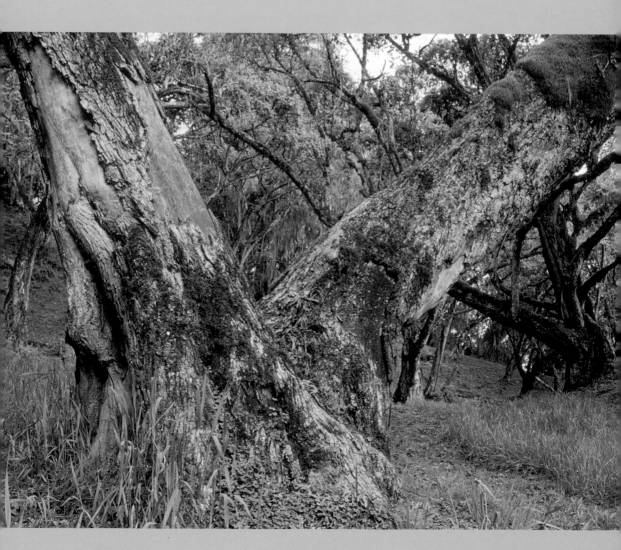

Traditional aromatherapy uses

Rosewood oil is traditionally used in aromatherapy for its sweet perfume in blends designed to uplift the mood, and in the beauty industry for its supposed skin-regenerating properties. It certainly has a soothing effect on the skin, and may be useful as a sweet-scented natural deodorant because of its mild antibacterial properties.

Ailments and remedies

Wrinkles and dry skin Use a blend of Rosewood and Jojoba oils as a nighttime moisturizer for wrinkles and mature skin. Add 1 drop of Rosewood oil to 1 teaspoon of Jojoba oil or vegetable oil, and massage gently into the face, neck, and chest (see Caution).

Emotional vulnerability Vaporize 3 drops of Rosewood oil in a vaporizer to help soothe feelings of emotional vulnerability, especially during times of change and stress. It can be blended with any of the other mood-uplifting oils, such as Bergamot, Mandarin, and Neroli.

Why it works

Linalool gives Rosewood oil its sweet floral aroma. It also has antibacterial properties. For some reason, in spite of linalool's reputation as a sedative, Rosewood oil is not usually thought of as a sedative. This is possibly because the linalool in Rosewood oil is a mixture of two chemical structures, whereas Lavender (*Lavandula angustifolia*, see page 102) only contains one structure of linalool.

Alpha-terpineol contributes to the antibacterial properties of the oil. Both linalool and alpha-terpineol may have mild cooling effects on the skin, which is possibly why it has been used in skin care.

Caution: If any irritation is caused, wipe off the skin and rinse with cold running water. It is unlikely, but some people have very sensitive facial skin.

Rosewood

Active constituents

linalool **85.3%**
alpha-terpineol **3.5%**

Other significant constituents

cis-linalool oxide **1.5%**
trans-linalool oxide **1.3%**
1,8-cineole **1%**
geranyl acetate **0.14%**

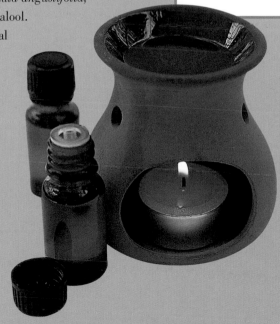

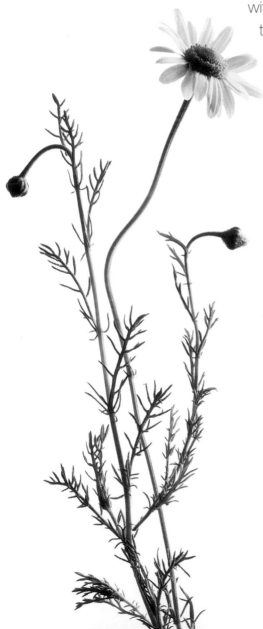

Anthemis nobilis, Chamaemelum nobile

Chamomile, Roman or English

Roman or English Chamomile has white daisy-like flowers with yellow centers and feathery leaves. It is thought that the name *chamomile* originates from the Greek words *kamai* (on the ground) and *melon* (apple), referring to the ground-creeping habit of the plant and its distinctive sweet apple-like odor.

The herb has been grown all over Europe for many centuries, cultivated for its calming effect on nervous disorders and its ability to alleviate depression. Some monastery healing gardens used to contain raised beds of *Anthemis nobilis*, so that convalescents staying at the monastery could lie on the plants and benefit from the odor released by crushing the plants. It seems that the plant thrives by being walked on, and some formal gardens have chamomile lawns especially for this purpose. The *Matricaria chamomilla* (German Chamomile, see page 106) plants are erect daisy-like bushes, and are thus easily distinguished from the creeping *A. nobilis*.

The oil of Roman Chamomile is produced by steam distillation of the flowers. It is pale yellow, occasionally tinged with blue, although the blue is never as intense as the blue of steam-distilled German Chamomile oil.

Traditional aromatherapy uses

Roman Chamomile oil is traditionally used as a relaxant and antidepressant. It has been used to reduce preoperative anxiety, and also to help relieve the mood swings associated with premenstrual syndrome (PMS). Some books state that it is as good an anti-inflammatory agent as German Chamomile oil, but there has yet to be an adequate controlled trial demonstrating this. The tea is given as an intestinal smooth-muscle relaxant, particularly suitable for colic in babies, but it remains to be seen whether this effect is due to the essential oil or to the water-soluble active principles.

Ailments and remedies

Nervous tension and anxiety Put 1 drop of Roman Chamomile oil on a tissue and tuck it into a shirt pocket or bra strap, so that the odor rises throughout the day. Alternatively, put 3 drops of Roman Chamomile oil into a vaporizer and vaporize for 2 hours in the bedroom before going to sleep, or in the place where the stressful situation occurs. Do not use the oil for more than a few days at a time, or the odor can become linked to the stressful situation itself and provoke the feelings of stress you are trying to alleviate.

Premenstrual syndrome (PMS) Add 3 drops of Roman Chamomile oil to 1 teaspoon of vegetable oil and massage gently into the abdomen and lower back, using soft clockwise circular strokes. Alternatively, run a warm bath (not too hot), and add 3 drops of Roman Chamomile oil to the water before getting into it. Allow the uplifting scent to ease away the irritability and stress.

Why it works

Isobutyl angelate is likely to be responsible for the oil's calming and anti-depressant effects. It is also gives the oil an apple-like odor.

2-methylbutyl angelate, methallyl angelate, isobutyl isobutyrate, and **isoamyl angelate** could contribute to Roman Chamomile's calming effects.

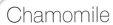

Chamomile

Active constituents

isobutyl angelate **35.9%**
2-methylbutyl angelate **15.3%**
methallyl angelate **8.7%**
isobutyl isobutyrate **4.9%**
isoamyl angelate **4.34%**

Other known constituents

pinocarvone **3.59%**

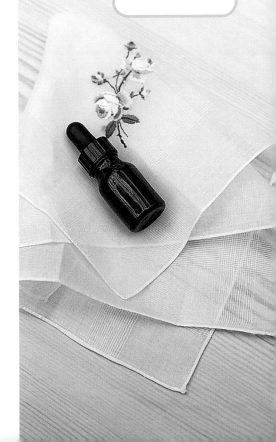

> Caution:
> Roman Chamomile oil should not be confused with
> Moroccan Chamomile oil (Ormenis mixta or O. multicola).
> Moroccan Chamomile oil is not often used in aromatherapy.

Boswellia carterii

Frankincense {Olibanum}

The oil of Frankincense is extracted from the resin of *Boswellia carterii* trees found in the desert areas of eastern Africa and the Arab peninsula. There are three *Boswellia* species that produce an essential oil-bearing resin: *B. carterii* (or sacra) (Arabic and Somalian), *B. frereana* (Somalian, Eritrean, Kenyan), and *B. serrata* (Indian).

Frankincense resin has been used since the times of the Egyptian pharaohs as an ingredient of medicines, cosmetics, and embalming mixtures. Cultures of the Middle East use the resin as an incense in religious ceremonies, and it is one of the components of the incense used by the Orthodox and Roman Catholic Churches. The tree naturally exudes the resin when the trunk is cut.

The essential oil of Frankincense is released from the resin by steam distillation, but can also be extracted by the CO_2 method.

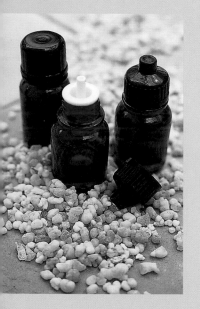

Traditional aromatherapy uses

Frankincense is used for wound healing and in beauty treatments for dry and aged skin, presumably because it has anti-inflammatory properties, and because it may stimulate cell regeneration. Frankincense oil shares astringent and mucous-drying properties with Cypress oil, and is useful for the treatment of congested respiratory diseases, including asthma.

Ailments and remedies

Dry skin and wrinkles Add 3 drops of Frankincense oil (either type) to 1 teaspoon of a skin-nourishing vegetable oil, such as Apricot Kernel oil, and massage gently into the face with short upward strokes, moving outward from the midline of the face. Add 1 drop of Rose oil to this blend for a special treat. Alternatively, make up a batch of cream, using 20 drops of Frankincense per 3 oz (100 g) of unscented base cream.

Stress-related shortness of breath and asthma If your breathing shortens when you are agitated or stressed, using Frankincense during meditation can accustom your body to relax whenever you smell Frankincense. Make time to sit in a dimly lit quiet room for 10 minutes, focusing on your breathing. Apply 2 drops of Frankincense oil directly to your collarbone as you sit, and let your breath become slow and even. Allow first your stomach muscles, and then all of your muscles, to relax.

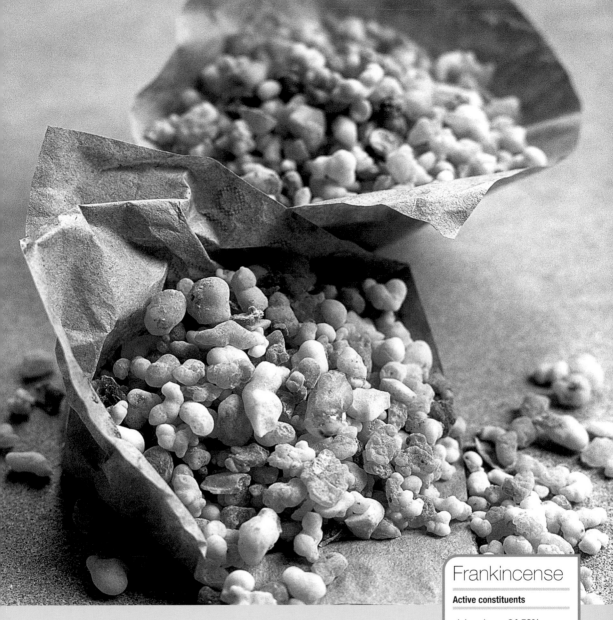

Why it works

There is some confusion about the chemical composition of Frankincense oil, but from the odor of the commonly available oil, it is likely to contain alpha-pinene, alpha-phellandrene, and para-cymene as major constituents.

Alpha-pinene helps break down excess mucous and contributes astringent properties, making the oil useful for treating congested respiratory diseases, including asthma.

Boswellic acids have been shown to have potent anti-inflammatory properties when taken orally.

Incensol and **incensyl acetate** contribute to the odor of Frankincense and are thought to make it helpful for prayer and meditation.

Frankincense

Active constituents

alpha-pinene **34.53%**
boswellic acids (major component of CO_2 extract, not present in steam-distilled oil)
incensol varies **<5%**
incensyl acetate varies **<2%**

Other known constituents

alpha-phellandrene **14.6%**
para-cymene **14%**
1,8-cineole **1%**
beta-bourbenene **0.32%**
beta-elemene **0.1%**
beta-caryophyllene **0.08%**
allo-aromadendrene **0.03%**

Cananga odorata var. genuina
Ylang ylang

Ylang ylang oil is extracted by steam distillation from the flowers of a tropical rainforest tree from the Annonaceae family, which is cultivated on several islands in the Indian Ocean. It probably originated in the Philippines, where the people would soak the fragrant yellow flowers in coconut oil and use the resultant heady lotion to perfume their hair and bodies.

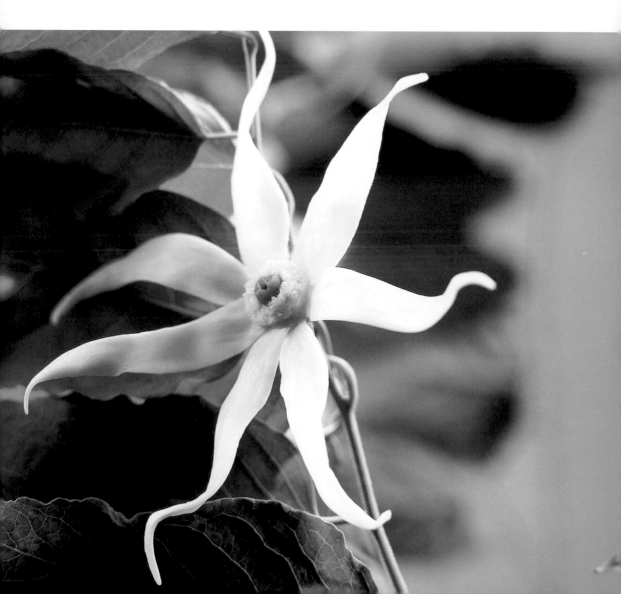

The odor is intensely sweet, with musky, earthy undertones. It is a smell that people almost always either love or hate. The extraction process is done in several fractions, because the most volatile compounds are the most prized in the perfumery industry, and the first fraction, known as Ylang ylang Super Extra, is much more expensive than the Extra, First, Second, or Third fractions, which are available in decreasing price order.

Traditional aromatherapy uses

Ylang ylang oil is most often recommended for sexual problems, especially lack of sexual desire. While it is not physiologically active in terms of creating a sexual response, its euphoric and relaxing properties probably help in setting the scene. Ylang ylang oil is also reputed to lower blood pressure and heartrate, and to act as an antispasmodic.

Ailments and remedies

Depressive moods or the "blues" To help alleviate blue moods, wear 1 drop of Ylang ylang as a perfume, either dabbed on your collarbone, or onto the inside front of your shirt, so that the aroma rises during the day. The oil is a little strong to vaporize continuously, so it is recommended to use it as a personal fragrance only.

Lack of sexual interest A full body massage with 5 drops of Ylang ylang in 2–3 tablespoons of vegetable oil is luxurious, and can lead to sensual lovemaking. Alternatively, a bath with three drops of Ylang ylang is relaxing and aphrodisiac.

Why it works

The various grades of Ylang Ylang oil vary in their chemical composition and use. The Super Extra grade contains the most para-cresyl methyl ether and linalool, and is prized for its euphoric fragrance. The Third grade Ylang ylang contains mainly anti-inflammatory molecules, such as beta-caryophyllene and farnesene. Most therapists prefer the "Complete" grade, which is a blend of all the different grades. This combines the euphoric and anti-inflammatory properties of the different constituents.

Linalool gives the oil sedative properties.

Beta-caryophyllene and **germacrene-D** may have possible anti-inflammatory properties.

Para-cresyl methyl ether contributes strong euphoric and heady qualities to the oil's aroma. It could also contribute antispasmodic effects.

Benzyl benzoate, geranyl acetate, benzyl acetate, and **benzyl salicylate** could contribute to the relaxing and calming effects of the oil.

Ylang ylang

Active constituents

linalool **19%**
beta-caryophyllene **10.5%**
germacrene D **10.2%**
para-cresyl methyl ether **8.7%**
benzyl benzoate **7.3%**
geranyl acetate **6.7%**
benzyl acetate **4.6%**
benzyl salicylate **2%**

Other significant constituents

farnesol **1.8%**
cadinols **1.8%**
eugenol **0.3%**
3-methyl-2-butenyl acetate **0.13%**
Various sesquiterpenes make up the rest of the oil

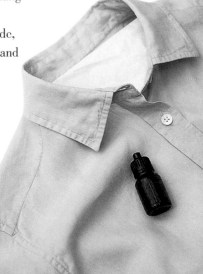

Canarium luzonicum
Elemi

Elemi oil is distilled from the oleoresin produced by *Canarium luzonicum*, a tropical tree indigenous to the Philippines. Elemi is from the Burseraceae family, as are Frankincense (*Boswellia carterii*) and Myrrh (*Commiphora myrrha*). The whitish oleoresin is exuded from the trunk and harvested when it has dried. The nuts of the tree are known as Manila or pili nuts, and contain nutritious protein and thick vegetable fat.

The oil is steam-distilled out of resin in a similar way to Frankincense. The Egyptians used Elemi resin in their embalming processes, but this may have come from other *Canarium* species. The powdered resin has been utilized as a healing agent for infected wounds, and is traditionally used in the Philippines to treat nonhealing ulcers. A species exists in Australia known as *C. muelleri*, the Queensland Elemi or Scrub Turpentine, which produces a resin with similar wound-healing properties. *C. schweinfurthii* is found in Africa, and also produces a resin, and edible nuts.

Traditional aromatherapy uses

Elemi oil is often used in conjunction with Frankincense oil, especially for the healing of wounds and skin infections. Both oils are also used to alleviate asthma, because they seem to have an anti-inflammatory effect on the bronchioles.

Ailments and remedies

Cuts and abrasions Add 5 drops of Elemi oil to a small bowl of water or saline (salt) solution. Squeeze a gauze in the solution. Apply to the cut and cover with a bandage.

Asthma For nighttime asthma, add 5 drops of Elemi oil to a vaporizer in the bedroom before going to sleep. Alternatively, put 2 drops of Elemi oil on the pillow, or onto the pajamas near the neck, so that the oil can diffuse upward during the night. Blend 5 drops of Elemi oil in 1 teaspoon of vegetable oil and massage it into the throat and upper chest in the morning to ease tightness of breath or feelings of congestion throughout the

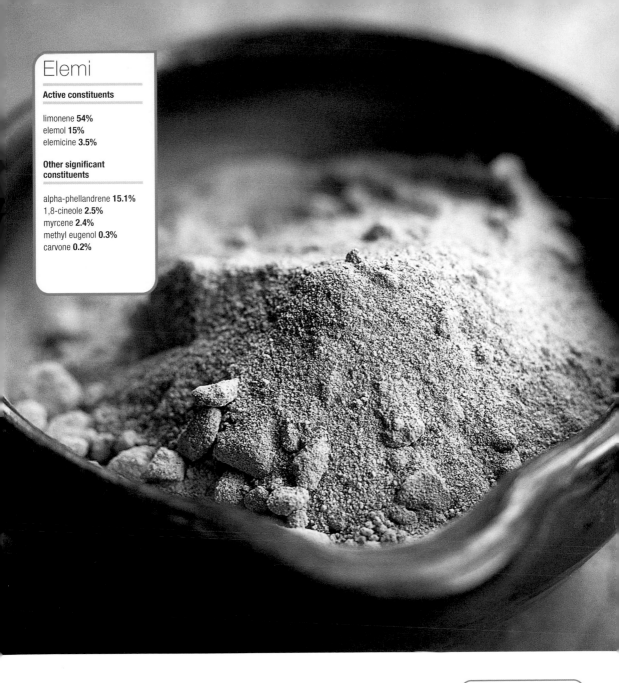

Elemi

Active constituents

limonene **54%**
elemol **15%**
elemicine **3.5%**

Other significant constituents

alpha-phellandrene **15.1%**
1,8-cineole **2.5%**
myrcene **2.4%**
methyl eugenol **0.3%**
carvone **0.2%**

day. The oil can be blended with Frankincense oil (but the total number of drops per teaspoon should not exceed 5).

Why it works

Limonene gives the oil its lemony smell, and in tests it shows promise as an antitumoral agent.

Elemol and **elemicine** give the oil its earthier, balsamic note, and may contribute to Elemi's uplifting and mild euphoric effects. It is also used as an ingredient of incense.

> **Caution:**
> It is important to store Elemi oil in cool, dark conditions because limonene can deteriorate easily. Old limonene may cause skin irritation in some people.

Cardamomum elettaria
Cardamom

Cardamom essential oil is extracted from the seeds of the Cardamom plant, also sometimes known as *Amomum elettaria*. The plant is from the Zingiberaceae family, like Ginger (*Zingiber officinalis*), but the rhizome (fleshy root) does not produce a commercial essential oil, as the rhizome of Ginger does. Cardamom's essential oil content is highest in the unripe seed pods, so they are harvested before ripening.

Cardamom is used as a spice in ayurvedic (traditional Hindu) medicine to counteract excesses of nervous energy and mucous in the lungs and digestive tract, and it is thought to increase "fire in the belly." It is an ingredient in the spiced Indian tea, chai, and one of the main components of the spice blend Garam Masala.

The fragrance of the oil is reminiscent of Eucalyptus, although it has a sweeter, earthier smell. Psychologically, the oil seems to open and widen the imagination, though it is not certain whether there are any constituents that are specifically psychotropic.

Traditional aromatherapy uses

Cardamom oil is a relative newcomer to aromatherapy, but it is being appreciated for its digestive-stimulant properties and its soothing effect on the lungs. It is used either in an abdominal massage, similarly to Fennel oil (*Foeniculum vulgare*, see page 90), or in combination with Eucalyptus oil (*Eucalyptus globulus*, see page 88) as an inhalation or as a foot rub.

Ailments and remedies

Flatulence Flatulence is often caused by the fermentation of partially digested proteins in the intestine. Tea brewed with a few cardamom seed pods can serve as a digestive aid after a heavy, meat-based meal (see Caution).

Coughs and colds Add 2 drops of Cardamom oil to a bowl of hot water for an inhalation to help loosen phlegm and soothe a dry cough. Add 1 drop of Cardamom oil and 2 drops of Sandalwood oil (*Santalum album*, see page 144) to 1 teaspoon of vegetable oil and externally anoint the throat with the blend to help soothe a sore throat.

Why it works

1,8-cineole gives Cardamom oil similar expectorant properties and odor to Eucalyptus (*Eucalyptus globulus*, see page 88) and Cajuput (*Melaleuca leucadendron*, see page 110) oils. Inhalation achieves the best effect.

Alpha-terpineol, linalool, terpinen-4-ol, and **geraniol** have broad-spectrum antibacterial properties. Combined with the 1,8-cineole, they make a good remedy for coughs and colds.

Caution: Do not take Cardamom essential oil internally (see *Eucalyptus globulus* Cautions, page 89).

Alpha-terpinyl acetate may contribute antispasmodic properties to the oil, making it useful for indigestion, and also to help release tightness in the chest.

Cardamom
Réunion Island

Active constituents

1,8-cineole **30.7%**
alpha-terpinyl acetate **30.6%**
alpha-terpineol **11.5%**
linalool **8.7%**
terpinen-4-ol **4.3%**
geraniol **1.4%**

Other known constituents

para-cymene **1.3%**
limonene **3.7%**
p-methylacetophenone **0.1%**
trans-carveol **0.1%**
trans-nerolidol **0.4%**

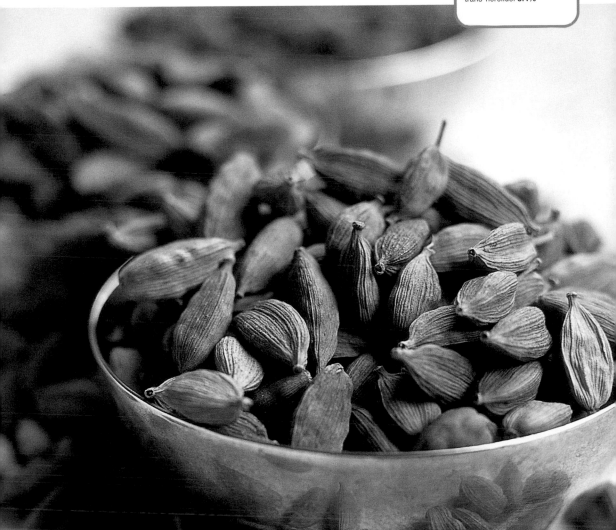

Citrus aurantium var. amara (flowers)

Neroli

Neroli is one of the most beautiful floral essential oils. It comes from the waxy white blossoms of the Bitter (or Seville) Orange tree, and is sometimes known as Orange Blossom oil. It is usually extracted by steam distillation, and the waters of distillation are used extensively in European and Arabian cooking—as are the waters from the distillation of Rose oil.

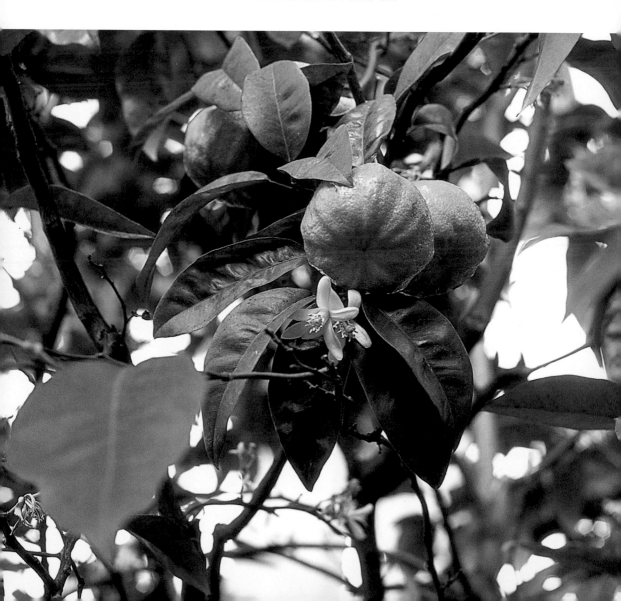

The name Neroli comes from the popularization of the oil by the Princess of Neroli during a plague in 17th-century Italy. The air in cities of the time was frequently foul from garbage in the streets and open sewers, and it was thought that the plague was transmitted through the air. The use of sweet-smelling flowers and perfumes was believed to ward off the infectious vapors, and it may well have contributed to the overall health of the people who could afford them. Orange blossoms are also traditionally used in bridal bouquets in Italy and Spain, their whiteness symbolizing purity, and their fragrance supposedly exerting a relaxing effect on nervous brides.

Traditional aromatherapy uses

Neroli oil is used primarily as an inhalation for depression and anxiety. It is also helpful in conditions where muscular spasm is associated with stress and anxiety, for example, in irritable bowel syndrome. Neroli oil is also used to treat skin affected by broken blood vessels and redness.

Ailments and remedies

Anxiety and stress Use the prediluted Neroli oil (3 percent in Jojoba oil), and wear it as a perfume for a week. If possible, learn a relaxation technique as well, so that you can associate a feeling of relaxation with the scent of the oil. Then, whenever you smell the oil, it will help you feel relaxed.

Intestinal spasms Either use the prediluted Neroli oil as above, or add 2 drops of pure Neroli oil to 1 teaspoon of vegetable oil. Massage it into the abdomen with gentle clockwise massage strokes, starting at the bottom of the belly on the person's left side.

Why it works

Linalool and **linalyl acetate** make up about a third of Neroli oil, and have a sweet floral scent and sedative properties. These compounds can help alleviate anxiety and nervous tension, like Lavender oil (*Lavandula angustifolia*, see page 102). Linalool may also contribute to Neroli's anti-inflammatory effects on the skin, making it useful in skin care.

Methyl N-methyl anthranilate, indole, and **cis-jasmone** are only present in small amounts in the oil, yet they are distinctive components of the oil's odor. They are also found in Jasmine oil (*Jasminum grandiflorum*, see page 94). These constituents may also contribute to Neroli and Jasmine oils' euphoric and antidepressant effects.

Caution: Neroli oil has a much lower limonene content than other citrus oils, but it is an expensive oil, so beware of immitations containing higher levels of limonene, as these could cause skin irritation.

Neroli

Active constituents

linalool **37.5%**
linalyl acetate **2.8%**
indole **0.1%**
methyl N-methyl anthranilate **0.1%**
cis-jasmone **0.05%**

Other significant constituents

limonene **16.6%**
beta-pinene **11.8%**
geraniol **4.25%**
nerolidol **2.6%**
geranyl acetate **1.7%**
neryl acetate **1%**
farnesol **0.9%**
terpinen-4-ol **0.75%**
alpha-terpinyl acetate **0.2%**

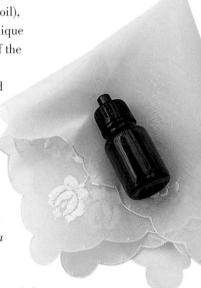

Citrus aurantium var. *amara* (leaves and twigs)
Petitgrain

Petitgrain oil is extracted by steam distillation from the leaves and twigs of the Bitter (or Seville) Orange tree, whose flowers yield Neroli oil. Petitgrain used to be distilled from the tiny unripe fruits, which were literally the *petits grains* (little grains). It is sometimes known as Bigarade oil, or *Citrus bigaradia*, and was first produced in France and Spain.

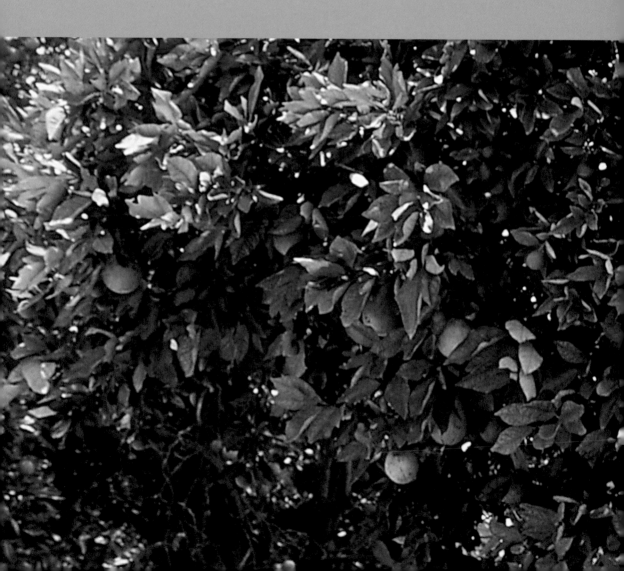

The oil is pale yellow, and has a characteristic woody green aroma, which also resembles the narcotic floral scent of the flowers. It bears little resemblance to the aroma of Orange-peel oil. Its primary use is in perfumery, and it was a base ingredient of many historic perfumes, notably the eau de Cologne made famous by Napoleon Bonaparte in the early 19th century. These days it is used in inexpensive fragrances, and in cosmetics and household products.

Traditional aromatherapy uses

Petitgrain oil is primarily viewed as a cheaper but harsher version of Neroli oil, though it is still used in skincare, particularly for acne and oily skin. It is also used to create a euphoric and relaxing blend for soothing anxiety and depression.

Ailments and remedies

Acne and oily skin Add 3 drops of Petitgrain oil to a bowl of warm water, squeeze a facecloth into the mixture, and press firmly into the face. Repeat as often as desired. It will have a mild astringent (drying) effect, so stop using it once the oiliness and acne are improving.

Why it works

Linalyl acetate and **linalool** have been shown to have sedative effects. They also occur in similar quantities in Bergamot (*Citrus bergamia*, see page 64), Lavender (*Lavandula angustifolia*, see page 102), and Neroli (*Citrus aurantium* var. *amara* flowers, see page 60) oils.

Alpha-terpineol and **linalool** both have soothing antibacterial properties, making the oil useful for acne and reddened skin.

Methyl N-methyl anthranilate (also found in Neroli oil, see page 60) is possibly responsible for the euphoric and mood-lifting effects of the oil, though the percentage varies.

Caution:

Do not use Petitgrain essential oil on the skin in conjunction with commercial acne preparations because it may cause irritation.

Petitgrain

Active constituents

linalyl acetate **45.5%**
linalool **24.1%**
alpha-terpineol **5.2%**
methyl N-methyl anthranilate **0.1%**

Other known constituents

geranyl acetate **4.2%**
limonene **4%**
neryl acetate **2.2%**
geraniol **1.8%**
beta-caryophyllene **1.6%**
nerol **8%**
2-phenylethanol **0.2%**
indole **0.05%**
2-methoxy-3-isobutyl pyrazine **0.01%**

Citrus bergamia

Bergamot

The lovely Bergamot flower may yield an essential oil, but it has not yet been extracted commercially.

Bergamot oil is derived from the Bergamot Orange (either *Citrus bergamia* or *C. aurantium* ssp. *bergamia),* grown in Italy for the purposes of essential-oil harvesting and candied preservation of the whole fruit. The area said to yield the best oil is Calabria in southern Italy. The oil is best known as the sweet, perfume-like flavoring in Earl Grey tea, or as an ingredient of eau de cologne.

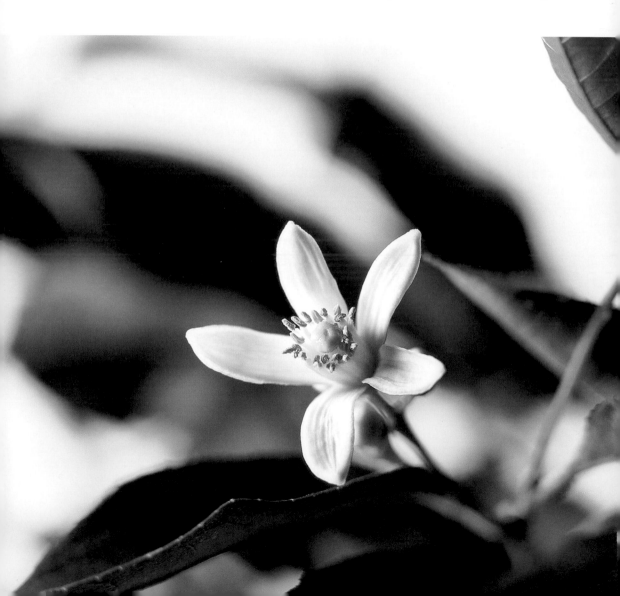

As in the other citrus fruits, the essential oil is found in little oil sacs embedded in the peel of the fruit. The best oil is produced by cold pressing (see page 15). The peel of the unripe fruit is crushed between two huge rollers, and the resulting oil collected. The oil is usually a pale greenish color.

Traditional aromatherapy uses

Bergamot oil is traditionally used as a mood lifter and as an antiseptic.

Ailments and remedies

Insomnia and nervous anxiety Run a deep warm bath at night (not too hot, or it will make you feel worse), light a candle, and switch off the light. Put 3 drops of Bergamot oil into the bath just before you get in, and swirl it around. If you prefer, add the oil to 1 tablespoon of powdered whole milk, which acts as an emulsifier, and then add it to the bath. The milk will also make your skin feel lovely and smooth. Stay in the bath for about 15 minutes, enjoying the vapors of the Bergamot oil, and letting yourself unwind.

Depressive moods The uplifting aroma of whole Bergamot oil may be helpful in alleviating the heaviness of depression. To prevent the oil from touching the skin, put 3 drops on a handkerchief and pin it to your clothes, so that your body warmth causes the oil to evaporate and bathe you in a cloud of beautiful scent during the day. Alternatively, put 3 drops in a vaporizer, or keep a small bottle of Bergamot oil in your pocket or at your desk, and just unscrew the lid when you need to change your mood.

Why it works

Limonene contributes to Bergamot oil's reputation as a digestive agent.
Linalyl acetate and **linalool** both have been shown to have sedative properties, and contribute to the oil's calming and anxiety-reducing effects.
Linalool is also an antibacterial agent.
Bergaptene is present in cold-pressed oil. It carries the distinctive Bergamot odor, but can cause skin reactions (see Caution). However, cold-pressed Bergamot oil can have the bergaptene removed by distillation.

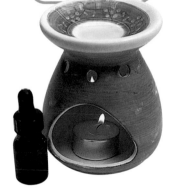

Bergamot

Active constituents

limonene **38.4%**
linalyl acetate **28%**
linalool **8%**
bergaptene **0.3%**

Other known constituents

gamma-terpinene **8%**
beta-pinene **7%**
aplha-pinene **1.4%**
sabinene **1.3%**
myrcene **1%**
geranyl acetate **0.5%**
geranial **0.4%**

Caution: There are no tests to prove that Bergamot oil has any antidepressant effects, so do not substitute for antidepressant medication.

Do not use cold-pressed Bergamot oil (especially if it is dark green in color: Rectified cold-pressed Bergamot oil is almost colorless) on the skin if it will be exposed to UV or sunlight within the next 12 hours. The combination of Bergamot oil and sunlight can cause redness, blistering, and development of an allergy known as Berloque dermatitis, which stains the skin brown.

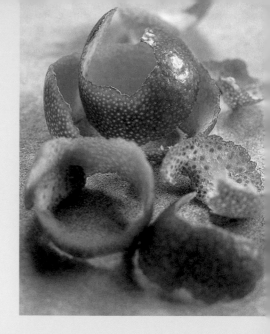

Citrus latifolia

Lime

Like Bergamot, Grapefruit, Lemon, Mandarin, Orange, and Tangerine oils, Lime essential oil is derived from the peel of citrus fruit. There are two kinds of lime: *Citrus latifolia* (known as Persian Lime), and *C. aurantifolia* (known as Key Lime). Lime juice is used in the cuisines of southern India, the Middle East, Southeast Asia, and the West Indies.

The juice was also used to prevent the Vitamin C deficiency disease known as scurvy, which affected the crews of sailing ships on long voyages. The leaves and twigs also produce an essential oil, which is similar in quality to the Petitgrain oil extracted from the leaves and twigs of Bitter Orange (*Citrus aurantium* var. *amara*, see page 60).

Lime oil can be extracted either by steam distillation or cold pressing, and the extraction processes influence the odor of the final product.

Caution: As with all citrus oils, storing Lime oil in the refrigerator will prolong its shelf life to 12 months. If stored at room temperature it should be disposed of after 6 months If you think the oil is old, do not use it on the skin. Do not use Lime oil in the bath as it can irritate delicate skin and mucous membranes.

Cold-pressed Lime oil has mild phototoxicity. Do not go out in the sun up to 12 hours after application of Lime oil to the skin.

Traditional aromatherapy uses

Lime oil of either species, both steam distilled and cold pressed, is traditionally used as an external disinfectant for cuts and stings, diluted by adding 1 or 2 drops to a bowl of clean water. Like Lemon oil, it is thought to be antiviral, particularly in aerosol form—although there have been no conclusive studies in this regard. Some sources claim that Lime oil can be used as an astringent in skincare preparations for oily skin, but it may be too irritating to the skin, so it should only be used in low concentrations for this purpose. The aroma of Lime oil is considered to be a stimulant and a refreshing tonic.

Ailments and remedies

Depressive moods or the "blues" Vaporize 3 drops of Lime oil in a vaporizer in the morning to give yourself a lift as you are waking up. Carry a small bottle of Lime oil with you during the day so as to inhale the aroma when your mood needs a lift.

Shaving rashes and acne Add 3 drops of Lime oil to a bowl of warm water.

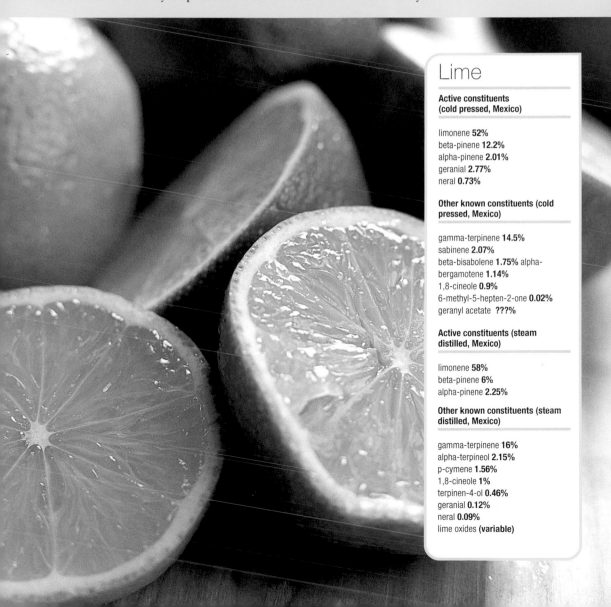
Squeeze a facecloth into the bowl and apply to the affected area. If there are distinct infected pimples, use a cotton swab to apply a tiny amount of Lime oil directly onto the pimple. The same procedure can be followed with Tea Tree oil (*Melaleuca alternifolia*, see page 108).

Why it works

Limonene has shown promise as an antitumor agent, and may help in the reduction of gall-bladder congestion. Citrus oils are used for poor digestion, and it is likely that the high limonene content is the active ingredient.

Alpha-pinene and **beta-pinene** have mild antibacterial properties.

Geranial and **neral** may help with acne due to their antibacterial activity.

Lime

Active constituents (cold pressed, Mexico)

limonene **52%**
beta-pinene **12.2%**
alpha-pinene **2.01%**
geranial **2.77%**
neral **0.73%**

Other known constituents (cold pressed, Mexico)

gamma-terpinene **14.5%**
sabinene **2.07%**
beta-bisabolene **1.75%** alpha-bergamotene **1.14%**
1,8-cineole **0.9%**
6-methyl-5-hepten-2-one **0.02%**
geranyl acetate **???%**

Active constituents (steam distilled, Mexico)

limonene **58%**
beta-pinene **6%**
alpha-pinene **2.25%**

Other known constituents (steam distilled, Mexico)

gamma-terpinene **16%**
alpha-terpineol **2.15%**
p-cymene **1.56%**
1,8-cineole **1%**
terpinen-4-ol **0.46%**
geranial **0.12%**
neral **0.09%**
lime oxides **(variable)**

Citrus limonum

Lemon

Lemon essential oil comes from the peel of citrus fruit, like Bergamot, Grapefruit, Lime, Mandarin, Orange, and Tangerine oils. It is used extensively for flavoring food and beverages, and was used in fragrancing detergents and other cleaning products, but these days synthetic lemon fragrances are preferred for their increased staying power and penetration.

Lemon juice has many more reported medicinal applications than Lemon oil—as an astringent and an antibacterial agent, for example. The antibacterial activity is probably responsible for the tradition of squeezing lemon juice onto seafood. Lemon juice is also supposed to be helpful in stopping bleeding, either from the nose or from wounds, though the acid of the juice would also sting. The seeds have been used to treat intestinal parasites, and a product known as Citricidin, made from various citrus seed extracts, can be used for amoebic infestations and worms.

The oil can be extracted either by steam distillation or by coldpressing, although cold pressing yields the more natural-smelling oil. It is not to be confused with lemon juice, and there is no Vitamin C or citric acid in Lemon oil. Both these substances come from the juice, not the peel. Some sources suggest that Lemon oil may be helpful internally in the management of blood-sugar levels in diabetes mellitus, but this has not yet been validated scientifically.

Traditional aromatherapy uses

Lemon is traditionally used in aromatherapy for its ability to uplift and focus the mind. It can also be used as an aerial disinfectant.

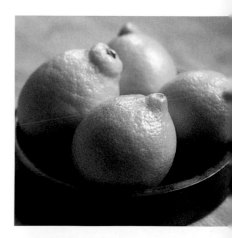

Ailments and remedies

Lack of focus and feeling "blue" Add 3 drops of Lemon oil to a vaporizer and diffuse into the air in the workspace. Alternatively, keep a bottle of Lemon oil on hand and inhale the aroma whenever you think the effect will be beneficial. This approach will also help disinfect the air in a closed workspace, and may increase productivity, as Japanese studies of Lemon oil have indicated.

Warts Use a clean cotton swab and dab undiluted Lemon oil onto the top of each wart. Repeat up to 6 times a day until the wart drops off. If possible, cover the wart with an adhesive bandage to aid penetration of the Lemon oil.

Why it works

Limonene may increase alertness.
Beta-pinene may contribute mild antiseptic effects.
Citral, **nonanal**, and **heptenal** may be antifungal agents.

Lemon

Main constituents

limonene **70%**
beta-pinene **11%**
citral **1.59**
nonanal **0.12%**
heptenal **0.02%**

Other known constituents

gamma-terpinene **8%**
geranyl acetate **0.22%**
trans-alpha-bergamotene **0.4%**

Caution:

Keep Lemon oil in the refrigerator to prolong its shelf life to a maximum of 12 months.

Do not use Lemon oil in the bath as it can irritate delicate skin and mucous membranes. If the oil irritates the skin, rinse off vigorously with running water.

Do not go out into the sun or UV light for 12 hours after applying cold-pressed Lemon oil to the skin.

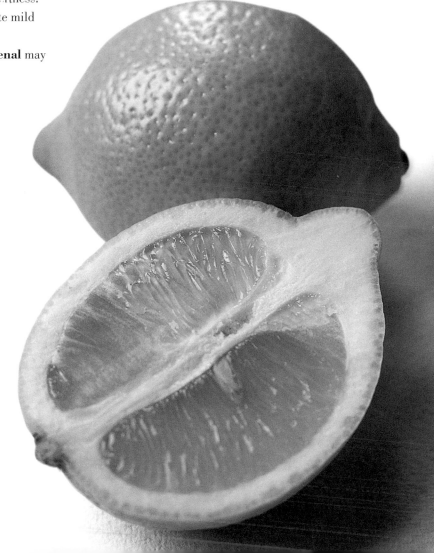

Citrus paradisii

Grapefruit

Grapefruit oil is another oil extracted from the peel of a citrus fruit. The fruit itself is a hybrid between the orange and a citrus known as *Citrus maxima*. Grapefruit is sometimes known as *C. racemosa*.

There are two varieties of Grapefruit that produce an essential oil: The thin-skinned, yellow-fleshed grapefruit, and the rosy-skinned, pink-fleshed grapefruit. As yet, no analysis of the two oils that shows any difference in constituents or odor.

The usual extraction process is cold pressing, in which the white lining of the fruit peel is first separated from the colored "flavedo," or flavored exterior. The flavedo is centrifuged to separate the oil from the solids. The solids can then be pressed for additional oil. The extracted oil is filtered and bottled.

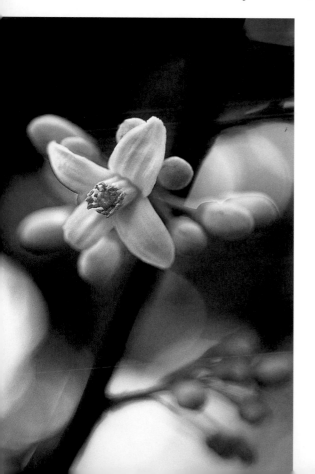

Traditional aromatherapy uses

Grapefruit oil is noted for its antidepressant and astringent properties, and is often used as a diuretic and for the treatment of cellulite.

Ailments and remedies

Swollen ankles Add 3 drops of Grapefruit oil to 1 tablespoon of vegetable oil and massage the affected ankle and leg with gentle squeezing strokes toward the heart. This encourages the lymph fluids to move, which can in turn help to reduce the swelling. You may need to be very gentle, because the swelling can be painful.

Cellulite Dilute the oil and apply as above. You can use stronger kneading strokes on the thighs and buttocks to get the cellulite moving.

Feeling "blue" Add 3 drops of Grapefruit oil to a vaporizer and experience the refreshing lift of the aroma. Add more drops as required, because the oil is volatile and will evaporate more quickly than other oils.

Why it works

Limonene is the major constituent in Grapefruit oil, and is responsible for the oil's citrus odor. In tests, limonene has shown promise as an antitumor agent, and may be helpful in improving bile flow. Limonene may also contribute to Grapefruit oil's diuretic properties, although other citrus oils high in limonene are not noted for a diuretic effect.

Nootkatone has a fresh, green, sour, fruity odor, and with the trace amounts of 1-p-menthene-thiol gives the unique grapefruity odor to the oil.

Octanal and **decanal** also contribute to the odor of the oil, and may irritate mucous membranes.

Grapefruit

Active constituents (Brazil)

limonene **93%**
nootkatone **0.3%**
octanal **0.29%**
decanal **0.27%**
1-p-menthene-thiol **(trace)**

Other known constituents (Brazil)

myrcene **1.97%**
alpha-pinene **0.59%**
beta-caryophyllene **0.3%**
linalool **<1%**

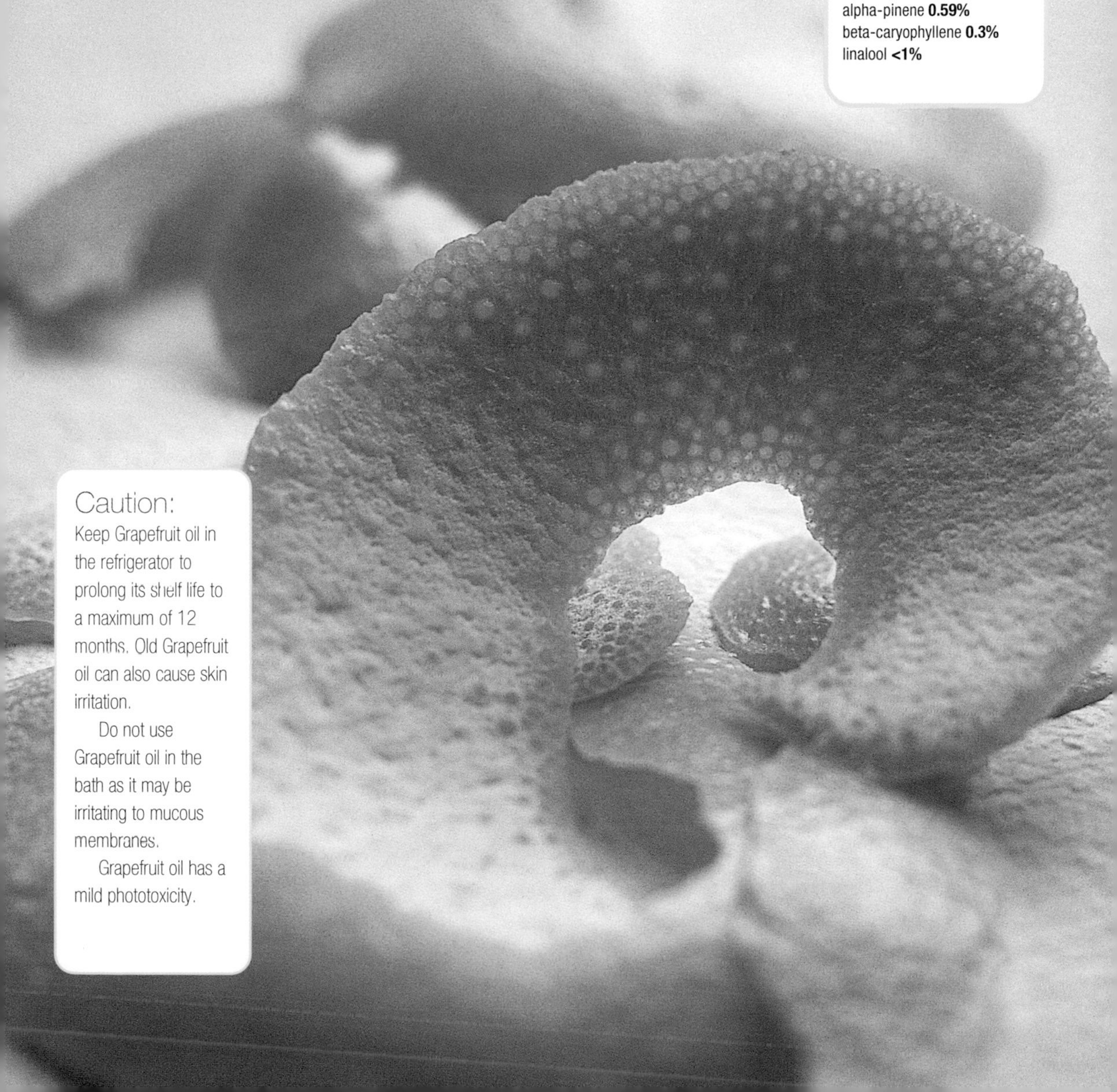

Caution:

Keep Grapefruit oil in the refrigerator to prolong its shelf life to a maximum of 12 months. Old Grapefruit oil can also cause skin irritation.

Do not use Grapefruit oil in the bath as it may be irritating to mucous membranes.

Grapefruit oil has a mild phototoxicity.

Citrus reticulata, C. deliciosa
Mandarin

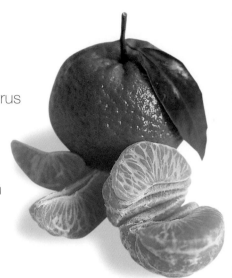

Mandarin essential oil is derived from the peel of citrus fruit, in the same way as Bergamot, Lemon, Lime, Orange, and Grapefruit oils. In China, where there are various cultivars available, the bright orange fruits are thought to bring good luck. In the northern hemisphere, they are traditionally associated with Christmas, because they are always imported from warmer climes at that time of year.

Mandarin oil is cold pressed from the ripe fruit peel, and is often a deep orange color, because some of the pigments from the peel come across in the process. It is the sweetest of the citrus oils and is known for its mood-lifting effects. The oil is used in flavoring drinks and confectionery. The high percentage of limonene makes it a likely digestive aid.

Traditional aromatherapy uses

Mandarin oil is widely considered to be one of the safest essential oils in aromatherapy, and is recommended by even the most cautious therapists for use during pregnancy and for the treatment of children. It is renowned as a mood-lifter, and also for helping to reduce anxiety.

Ailments and remedies

Depressive moods or the "blues" Vaporize 3 drops of Mandarin oil in a vaporizer to relax and enliven you. Carry a small bottle of Mandarin oil around with you, so that you can inhale it whenever you need cheering.

Irritable or overtired children Vaporize 3 drops of Mandarin oil in a vaporizer in the child's bedroom, or put 1 drop of Mandarin oil on the child's pajamas. The aroma should help settle an irritable child—but check first that the child likes the smell!

Low energy and jet lag Put 3 drops of Mandarin oil into a bowl of warm water and squeeze a facecloth into it. Press the warm cloth into your face and inhale the delicious aroma, breathing deeply to revitalize yourself. Repeat until you feel reenergized. This is also a refreshing tonic before going to a party, or during long-haul airplane travel. As always, it is

Caution: As with all citrus oils, keep Mandarin oil in the refrigerator to prolong its shelf life. If you have had the bottle for more than 12 months, or it smells at all pine-like, do not use it on the skin because the deteriorated products may cause skin sensitization.

important to consult a doctor or naturopath if the low energy levels persist and the fatigue continues for more than two weeks without obvious cause.

Why it works

Limonene is responsible for Mandarin oil's citrus odor. In tests, limonene has shown promise as an antitumor agent, and may also be helpful in the reduction of gall-bladder congestion.

Methyl N-methyl anthranilate gives Mandarin oil its characteristic odor, and may be the compound responsible for its mood-lifting effects. This compound is also found in Jasmine (*Jasminum grandiflorum*, see page 94), Neroli (*Citrus aurantium* var. *amara*, see page 60), and Sweet Orange oils (*Citrus sinensis*, see page 74) in small quantities.

Mandarin
Italy (cold pressed)

Active constituents

limonene **71%**
methyl N-methyl anthranilate **0.15%**

Other known constituents

gamma-terpinene **18.54%**
alpha-pinene **2.39%**
alpha-sinensal **0.2%**
octanal **0.17%**
decanal **0.07%**
nonanal **0.07%**

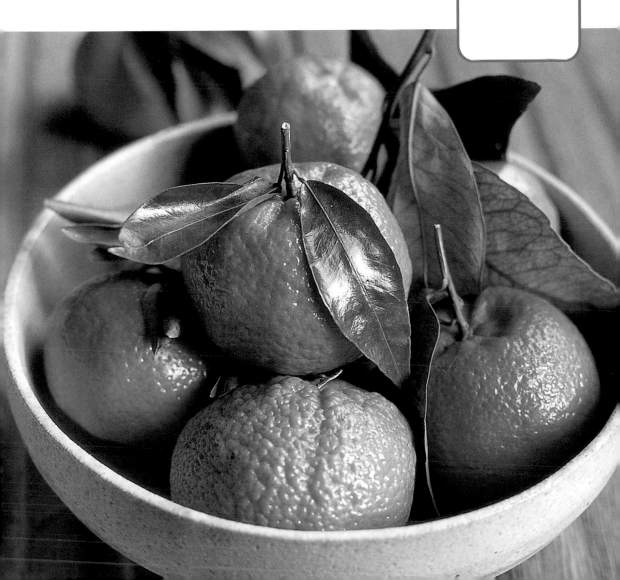

Citrus sinensis

Sweet Orange

Sweet Orange oil is extracted from the ripe fruit peel of *Citrus sinensis*. Sweet Oranges have been recognized as a valuable food source for centuries, in both Western and Eastern cultures. The fruit is a good source of Vitamin C, but the essential oil contains none. In China, a gift of oranges is considered a harbinger of good fortune, because of the fruit's golden color, which is said to symbolize wealth. Sweet Orange oil is cold pressed and is usually pale yellow. It is most similar to Mandarin oil (*Citrus reticulata*, see page 72).

Caution: Sweet Orange oil should not be confused with oil from the peel of Bitter Orange (*Citrus aurantium*), which is likely to contain more of the furocoumarins that can cause photosensitization on the skin in sunlight.

Keep Sweet Orange oil in the refrigerator to prolong its shelf life to a maximum of 12 months.

Do not use Sweet Orange oil in the bath as it can cause irritation to sensitive skin and mucous membranes.

Traditional aromatherapy uses

Like Mandarin oil, Sweet Orange oil is often used as an antidepressant. It is reputed to be useful in stimulating appetite, and may be helpful in the management of anorexia nervosa. Some sources suggest that it is also useful as a diuretic in reducing cellulite.

Ailments and remedies

Depressive moods or the "blues" Vaporize 3 drops of Sweet Orange oil in a vaporizer to help lift the spirits. Make an enlivening Sweet Orange spritz by adding 3 drops of Sweet Orange oil to 1 pint (500 ml) of filtered water. Decant the spritz into an atomizer or spray bottle. Shake well before use, and keep your eyes closed when you spritz.

Lack of appetite Vaporize 3 drops of Sweet Orange oil in the dining room

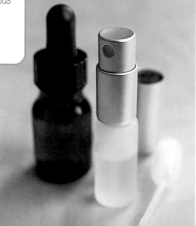

or kitchen area while you are preparing food. The sweet smell may help to stimulate your salivary juices.

Cellulite Add 3 drops of Sweet Orange oil to 1 tablespoon of vegetable oil and gently massage the legs with small circular movements upward from ankle to thigh. This should get the lymph fluids moving, and help reduce cellulite.

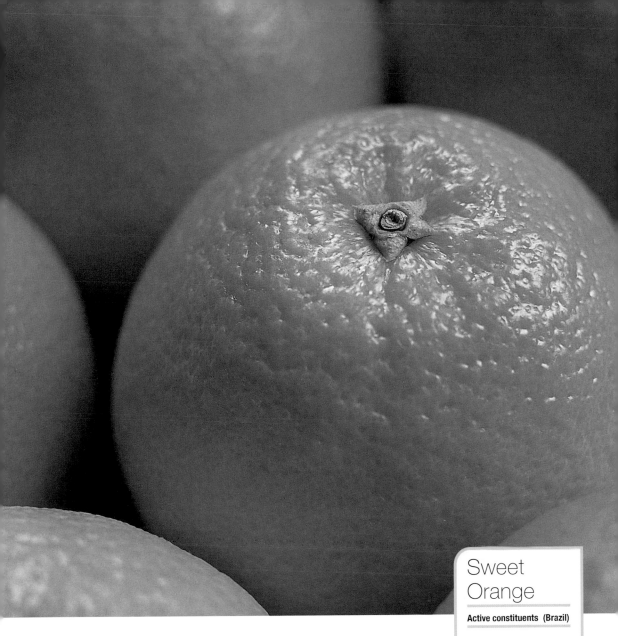

Sweet Orange

Active constituents (Brazil)

limonene **89%**
auraptene **0.09%**
methyl N-methyl anthranilate
(less than 1%)
bergamottin **(trace)**

**Other known constituents
(Brazil)**

myrcene **1.71%**
beta-bisabolene **1.29%**
1-nonanol **0.67%**
linalool **0.35%**
neral **0.25%**
decanal **0.2%**
geranial **0.19%**
linalyl acetate **0.14%**

Why it works

Limonene is the major constituent in Sweet Orange oil, and is responsible for the oil's citrus odor. In tests, limonene has shown promise as an antitumor agent, and may help in reducing gall-bladder congestion. Sweet Orange oil's reputation as a digestive aid may come from its limonene content.

Methyl N-methyl anthranilate gives Sweet Orange oil its characteristic sweet fruity smell, and may be the compound in the oil responsible for its mood-lifting effects.

Auraptene and **bergamottin** are two components which may cause photosensitization, and should be well below 1% in the oil if it is to be used on the skin. This is normally the case, especially with steam-distilled oils.

Commiphora myrrha, C. molmol
Myrrh

Myrrh resin comes from cuts made in the bark of *Commiphora myrrha* trees of the Burseraceae family, and is a close cousin of Frankincense (*Boswellia carterii*) and Elemi (*Canarium luzonicum*). Myrrh is used as an incense across the Arab world, and is also found in most church incense mixtures.

The antibacterial and wound-healing properties of powdered Myrrh resin have been known for centuries. The ancient Egyptians used it in their embalming mixtures, and in their cosmetic preparations and perfumes. In ayurvedic medicine, myrrh resin is used in the treatment of heart disease, and may help prevent blood clots. A decoction of the resin is used as a gargle for infections of the mouth and gums. Preliminary research into the anti-inflammatory properties of Myrrh resin shows great promise for its use in irritable bowel syndrome. The essential oil probably does not have the same properties, because steam-distillation is not effective in extracting large compounds. The Myrrh oil used in aromatherapy is a steam extraction of the resin, which yields a thick, reddish-brown oil with a distinctive balsamic resinous odor.

Traditional aromatherapy uses
Myrrh is considered an oil for the skin and is effective in treating wounds, pimples, or boils. It is also used to clear mucous in respiratory infections.

Ailments and remedies
Cuts and abrasions Add 5 drops of Myrrh oil to a bowl of clean, warm water. Squeeze a gauze dressing into the solution and use it to wipe the cut. Alternatively, put undiluted Myrrh oil onto the skin around a large cut, or directly onto a scratch.

Wrinkles Add 1 drop of Myrrh oil to 1 teaspoon of Jojoba oil and apply to wrinkles of the face and neck, avoiding the eyes. This is best done at nighttime, to allow the oil ample time to soak into the skin.

Pimples Dab pimples directly with a cotton swab dipped in Myrrh. Repeat two times a day.

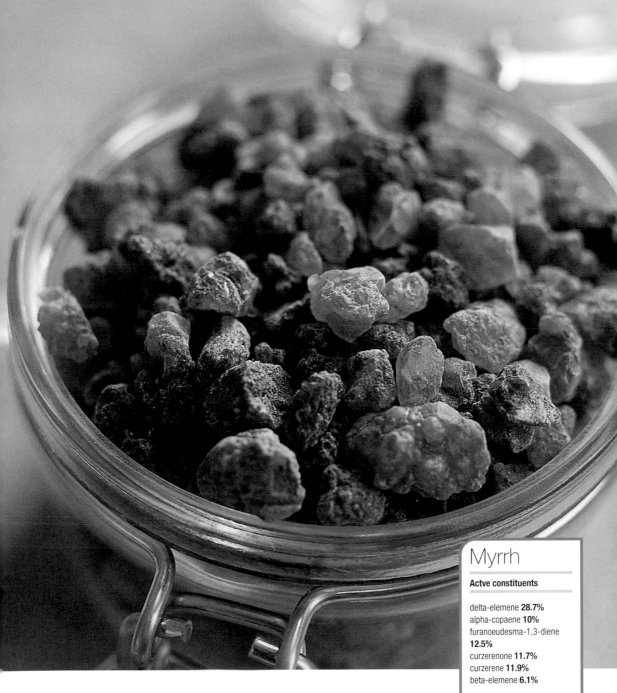

Why it works

Delta-elemene, alpha-copaene, beta-elemene, and **curzerene** are likely to contribute to Myrrh oil's anti-inflammatory properties. The element compounds have antitumor properties and may also help to lower cholesterol, but the evidence is inconclusive.

Furanoeudesma-1,3-diene and **curzerenone,** and the furans and furfurals contribute to Myrrh's distinctive odor, and probably also to its anti-inflammatory and wound-healing properties.

Myrrh

Actve constituents

delta-elemene **28.7%**
alpha-copaene **10%**
furanoeudesma-1,3-diene **12.5%**
curzerenone **11.7%**
curzerene **11.9%**
beta-elemene **6.1%**

Other known constituents

methyl isobutyl ketone **5.6%**
2-methyl-5-isopropenyl furan **4.6%**
lindestrene **3.5%**
3-methyl-2-butenal **2.2%**
dihydrocurzerenone **1.1%**
assorted furans, furfurals

Coriandrum sativum

Coriander

Coriander is a herb from the Umbelliferae family, also known as cilantro. It has leaves like those of Mediterranean parsley, and is used in Mexican, Indian, Vietnamese, and Thai cuisine. The umbrella-shaped flowerheads have a pale purple hue, and produce little round fruits which are used as a spice in Indian and Middle Eastern cookery.

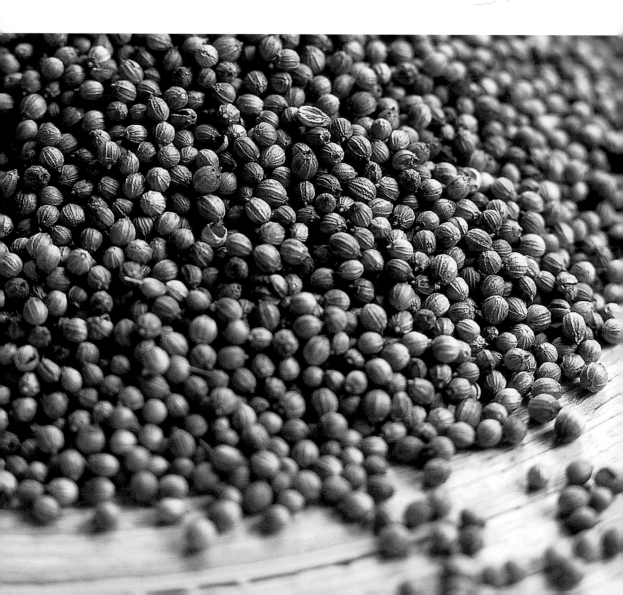

The pale yellow essential oil used in aromatherapy is extracted by steam distillation from powdered dried fruits that have developed the desired aroma. Fresh fruits smell more like the leaf, which is not an especially pleasant scent for aromatherapy purposes. As with many of the seed oils from the Umbelliferae family—such as Sweet Fennel (*Foeniculum vulgare* var. *dulce*, see page 90) and Aniseed (*Pimpinella anisum*, see page 130)—Coriander oil is thought to aid digestion.

Traditional aromatherapy uses

In Indian traditional medicine, Coriander fruits are used to reduce excess heat in the body. Because of the spice's reputation as a digestive aid, Coriander oil is mostly used for colic, heartburn, and flatulence. Some sources suggest that the oil helps relieve rheumatic pain.

Ailments and remedies

Rheumatic pain Add 5 drops of Coriander oil to 1 tablespoon of vegetable oil and massage gently into the affected area. Repeat as necessary. Alternatively, blend 3 drops of Coriander oil with 1 drop of Lavender oil (*Lavandula angustifolia*, see page 102) and 1 drop of German Chamomile oil (*Matricaria chamomilla*, see page 106).
Indigestion and colic Add 3 drops of Coriander oil to 1 tablespoon of vegetable oil and massage the abdomen in gentle clockwise circles, starting at the person's bottom right-hand side.

Why it works

Linalool is the major component of Coriander oil, and probably accounts for the relaxant effect on the digestive system and the relief of rheumatic pain. It may also have a sedative effect generally, although it is not noted for this in aromatherapy.
Limonene is thought to help promote bile flow, although in these smaller amounts it is unlikely to contribute much to these properties in the oil.

Camphor has bloodflow-stimulating properties in low amounts, and could contribute to the use of the oil in rheumatism.

Coriander
Active constituents
linalool **69.4%**
limonene **6.2%**
camphor **4.1%**
Other known constituents
para-cymene **3.8%**
alpha-pinene **3.4%**
1,8-cineole **1.8%**
geraniol **1%**
2-decenal **(trace)**

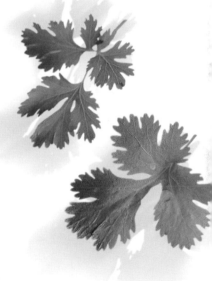

Caution: Do not use the less common, dark-green Coriander leaf oil on the skin. It could cause irritation due to its 2-decenal content.

Cupressus sempervirens

Cypress

The Cypress oil that is used in the perfumery industry derives from the *Cupressus sempervirens* tree, although there are several other species of *Cupressus* that produce a volatile oil. Some *Juniperus* species are also known as cypress trees, and there is sometimes confusion with the various cedar species. The Australian Blue Cypress oil comes from the heartwood of *Callitris intratropica*, but bears no similarity to the needle oil produced from *C. sempervirens*.

Cypress

Active constituents

alpha-pinene **47.9%**
delta-3-carene **19.8%**
cedrol **6.8%**
alpha-terpinenyl acetate **1.7%**
bornyl acetate **0.4%**

Other significant constituents

limonene **4.1%**
delta-cadinene **0.3%**
sabinene **1.17%**

The oil is extracted from the leaves and woody fruits by steam distillation, and is distinguished from Pine oil by its fresh and woody odor, in contrast to the "medicinal" smell of Pine oil.

The alcoholic tincture of Cypress is used for menstrual problems, including hot flashes during menopause, and some sources suggest that the oil has similar properties, although no testing has been done in this area.

Traditional aromatherapy uses

Cypress oil is used in aromatherapy as an astringent and as a diuretic. An astringent literally means "an agent that causes drying," and the oil is used to tighten and tone up loosened tissues. Cypress oil may be helpful in the temporary relief of hemorrhoids. It is also useful in cases of cellulite. As with Pine oil, the constituents are readily excreted in the urine, which causes a diuretic effect.

Ailments and remedies

Hemorrhoids Add 3 drops of Cypress oil to a shallow warm bath and sit or kneel in the bathtub, gently swooshing the affected area with the water. Repeat two or three times a day, if possible. Alternatively, add 20 drops of Cypress oil to a 3-oz (100-g) jar of unscented base cream. Apply to the affected area as often as needed. As always, consult your doctor for serious health complaints.

Cellulite and swollen ankles Add 10 drops of Cypress oil to 2 tablespoons of vegetable oil (use one half on each leg or arm). Apply the oil to the limb after a warm bath, starting at the extremity and moving up toward where the

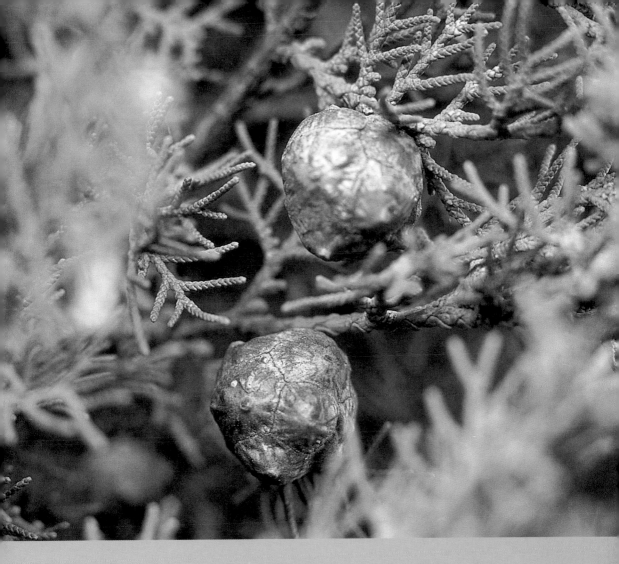

limb joins the body. Use little gentle squeezing strokes upward. Work toward the heart, so that you don't force the valves in the veins back the wrong way.

Why it works

Alpha-pinene contributes to Cypress oil's stimulating properties. It also helps to break down mucous and probably contributes to the vasoconstrictive effects along with cedrol.

Cedrol may have an anti-inflammatory effect, which would help with hemorrhoids.

Delta-3-carene on its own as a chemical can cause possible skin allergies. In combination with the other components of Cypress oil it does not appear to cause this problem. Content of delta-3-carene varies with different oil sources, so if concerned, ask your supplier.

Alpha-terpinyl acetate and **bornyl acetate** impart a freshness to Cypress oil that distinguishes it from the otherwise chemically similar Pine (*Pinus sylvestris*) oil.

> ## Caution:
> Do not use Cypress oil on sensitive skin, or if you have skin allergies due to possible sensitization by delta-3-carene (see Why it works).
>
> Avoid direct massage of varicose veins.

Cymbopogon citratus
Lemongrass

Lemongrass oil is extracted by steam distillation from the leaves of *Cymbopogon citratus,* also known as *Citratus flexuosus*, a tropical grass that grows widely in Southeast Asia, and is used as a flavor ingredient in savory dishes throughout the region. It is particularly distinctive in Thai cuisine, where its fragrant lemony flavor blends well with coconut milk.

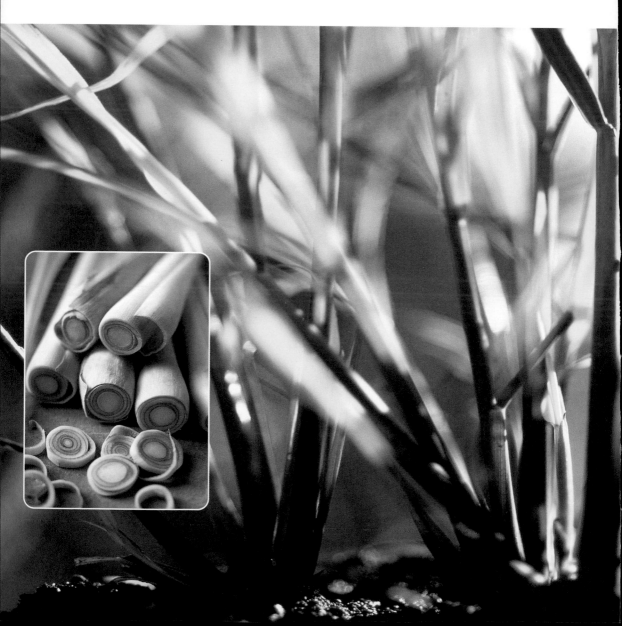

There are several oil-producing species of Cymbopogon, two of which are also produced commercially: Palmarosa (*C. martinii*, see page 84) and Citronella (*C. winterianus*, see page 86).

Lemongrass oil is less volatile than Lemon oil and does not oxidize as rapidly, so it is more useful in commercial preparations that need a long shelf life. The oil is thought to repel mosquitoes and flies.

Traditional aromatherapy uses

Lemongrass oil is used as a topical antiseptic and antifungal agent. It is thought to be a warming remedy for aching muscles and joints. The odor is stimulating and invigorating, and could be used for sluggish circulation and low energy.

Ailments and remedies

Athlete's foot (tinea) Add 3 drops of Lemongrass oil and 3 drops of Tea Tree oil (*Melaleuca alternifolia*) to a footbath or bowl of warm water, and let the feet or other affected part stay in the water for 5–10 minutes. After bathing, dry the affected area with a clean towel. With a clean cotton swab, apply undiluted Lemongrass oil directly to the infected area. Cover with an adhesive bandage, and repeat the process 2–3 times a day until the infection is clear. If the undiluted oil stings too much, add 10 drops of Lemongrass oil to a teaspoon of vegetable oil and use that instead.

Low energy or tiredness Add 3 drops of Lemongrass oil to 1 tablespoon of vegetable oil and massage into your calves and feet, using strokes that move up the legs toward the heart. You can do the same with the arms. You can also vaporize 3 drop of Lemongrass oil for an invigorating effect.

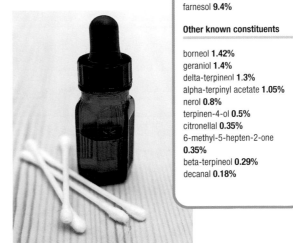

Lemongrass
India

Active constituents

geranial **48.15%**
neral **31.3%**
farnesol **9.4%**

Other known constituents

borneol **1.42%**
geraniol **1.4%**
delta-terpineol **1.3%**
alpha-terpinyl acetate **1.05%**
nerol **0.8%**
terpinen-4-ol **0.5%**
citronellal **0.35%**
6-methyl-5-hepten-2-one **0.35%**
beta-terpineol **0.29%**
decanal **0.18%**

Why it works

Neral and **geranial** when present together in an oil are jointly known as Citral. The oil's antifungal properties are attributed to **Citral**, and probably its stimulating and insect repellant effects also.

Farnesol has been shown to kill leukemia cells in the laboratory, and may show this activity in further clinical tests. Farnesol also has antibacterial properties, as do the minor constituents found in the oil.

> ### Caution:
> Lemongrass can irritate sensitive skin. Always dilute Lemongrass oil in vegetable oil, and avoid using it in the bath or in face preparations.

Cymbopogon martinii

Palmarosa

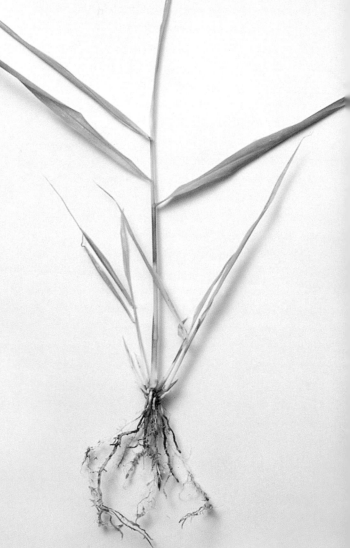

Palmarosa oil is extracted from one of a group of fragrant grasses that grow in the tropical areas of Southeast Asia. The other grasses, Lemongrass (*Cymbopogon citratus*) and Citronella (*C. winterianus*), have a strong lemony scent and are useful as insect repellents, whereas Palmarosa is less effective for this purpose. Unlike Lemongrass, Palmarosa stems are not used in cooking.

Palmarosa has been harvested commercially as a source of geraniol—also the main component of Geranium oil (*Pelargonium graveolens*, see page 128)—and as a starting ingredient for other fragrance materials since the early 19th century. The oil is extracted by steam distillation and is pale yellow, with a sweet, geranium-like smell.

Traditional aromatherapy uses

Palmarosa oil is often used for similar purposes to Geranium and Rose oil (*P. graveolens* and *Rosa damascena*, see pages 128 and 138), particularly for skincare, where it is thought to aid dry skin and skin rejuvenation. It is also useful as a natural deodorant, because its antibacterial properties kill the bacteria that cause the odor, and its geranium smell is not too strong.

Ailments and remedies

Dry skin and wrinkles Cleanse the face, using either hot water and a facecloth or a commercial skin cleanser. Add 3 drops of Palmarosa oil to 1 teaspoon of vegetable oil, and gently massage into the face and neck with your fingertips. This can be done either at night or during the day, since the oil does not contain any photosensitizing compounds.

Unpleasant body odor Really unpleasant body odor can be caused by various metabolic imbalances, so if it persists for more than a couple of weeks, consult a doctor or a naturopath. To prevent normal body odor, first wash the armpits with a rough cloth. For best results, omit the use of soap or detergent, because the lipids in the soap seem to feed the bacteria. Thoroughly dry your armpits, then drop 2–3 drops of Palmarosa oil into your palms, rub them together, and apply the oil to your armpits using your hands. Men may like to add another oil, such as Sandalwood or Cedarwood, for a more masculine smell, but Palmarosa oil tends to have "unisex" appeal.

Why it works

Geraniol has marked antibacterial and antifungal properties, and in combination with **linalool** and **farnesol** gives the oil its antibacterial properties. Body odor is partly caused by skin bacteria, so Palmarosa oil can help prevent body odor.

Geraniol, **geranyl acetate**, and **geranyl butyrate** give Palmarosa oil its geranium-like odor. **Geranyl acetate** may contribute mild antispasmodic properties to the oil.

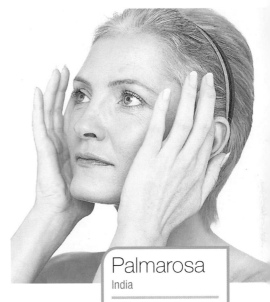

Palmarosa
India

Active constituents

geraniol **80%**
geranyl acetate **8.25%**
linalool **2.79%**
farnesol **1%**
geranyl butyrate **0.15%**

Other significant constituents

beta-caryophyllene **1.76%**
neral **0.4%**
alpha-farnesene **0.25%**
gamma-selinene **0.24%**

Cymbopogon winterianus

Citronella

Citronella oil is produced from two species of aromatic grass that grow in many parts of Southeast Asia. The two main production areas are Sri Lanka and Java. The Sri Lankan Citronella (*Cymbopogon nardus*) oil is preferred in perfumery for its rose-like odor. The Java Citronella oil (*C. winterianus*), on the other hand, has the characteristic lemon odor associated with Citronella candles and insect-repellent sprays.

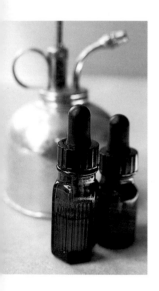

Other oils from the *Cymbopogon* genus include Lemongrass (*C. citratus* or *C. flexuosus*) and Palmarosa (*C. martinii*), and both are used in aromatherapy for different purposes (see preceding entries). The oils are extracted by steam distillation, and the choice of Citronella oil is a matter of personal preference. The more lemony Java oil is likely to be a better insect repellent.

Traditional aromatherapy uses

Citronella oil is traditionally used as an insect repellent, for mosquitoes and sandflies, and also fleas. It can be vaporized, or sprayed onto the bedding of pets (who probably won't like the smell). Some pet shampoos contain Citronella oil. Given the chemical composition of the oil, it could well be used in combination with other oils, such as Tea Tree (*Melaleuca alternifolia*), as an antibacterial agent. The lemony-rosy aroma is milder than Lemongrass and makes a pleasant-smelling blend.

Ailments and remedies

Insect repellent Add 3 drops of Citronella oil (either type) to a 2-pint (1-liter) spray bottle, and shake vigorously. Spray on limbs, clothing, and hats to repel mosquitoes and flies. Reapply whenever necessary. Alternatively, add 5 drops of Citronella oil to a vaporizer and position it close to where you are sitting. If the odor becomes too strong, stop vaporizing.

Caution:

Avoid contact with the eyes. If it does get into the eyes, wipe with a clean tissue toward the nose, and then splash with cold running water and wipe until the irritation subsides.

It is best to avoid using Citronella in the bath because it can be irritating to delicate areas.

Do not rely on Citronella oil for protection against mosquito bites in malaria-infested areas. It is advisable to wear long pants and sleeves in malarial areas, and not to go out at dusk when mosquitoes are biting.

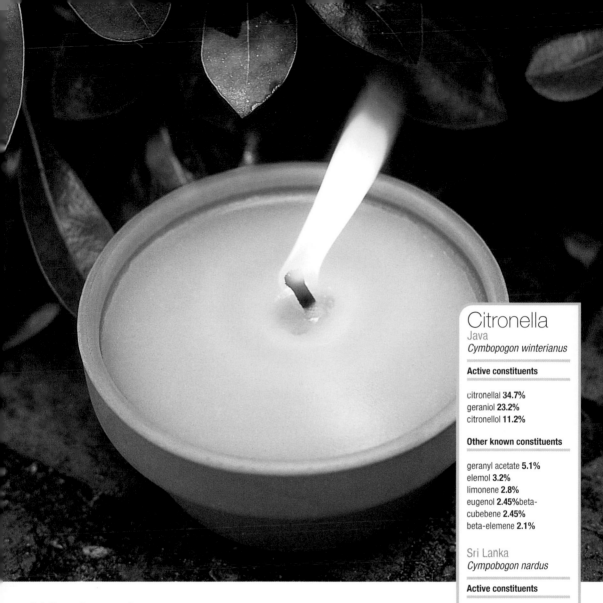

Citronella

Java
Cymbopogon winterianus

Active constituents

citronellal **34.7%**
geraniol **23.2%**
citronellol **11.2%**

Other known constituents

geranyl acetate **5.1%**
elemol **3.2%**
limonene **2.8%**
eugenol **2.45%**beta-
cubebene **2.45%**
beta-elemene **2.1%**

Sri Lanka
Cympobogon nardus

Active constituents

geraniol **18%**
citronellol **8.4%**
methyl isoeugenol **7.2%**
borneol **6.6%**
citronellal **5.2%**

Other known constituents

camphene **8%**
limonene **9.7%**
geranyl formate **4.2%**
beta-carophyllene **3.2%**
alpha-pinene **2.6%**
citronellyl acetate **1.9%**
elemol **1.7%**
methyl eugenol **1.7%**
geranyl butyrate **1.5%**

Why it works

Geraniol contributes the rose-like aroma to Sri Lankan Citronella oil, although both types have the lemon scent that comes from **citronellol** and **citronellal**. All three compounds also have antibacterial properties, which are enhanced by the presence of eugenol in the Java Citronella oil.

Citronellal may cause irritation on sensitive skin, although it is probably the agent in the oil that gives it its insect-repellent effects.

Methyl isoeugenol in Sri Lankan Citronella oil may contribute an uplifting effect.

Borneol gives Sri Lankan Citronella oil a camphoraceous note, which may also contribute to the insect-repellent effects.

Eucalyptus globulus

Eucalyptus

There are over 500 species of Eucalyptus indigenous to Australia, and several of these were cultivated in other countries, such as China, Spain, and South Africa for their fast-growing timber and their yield of commercially useful essential oils. *Eucalyptus globulus* is the Eucalyptus oil most commonly used in aromatherapy. *E. radiata* is similar in odor. The oil is extracted by steam distillation from the leaves and twigs.

Eucalyptus
Spain

Active constituents

1,8-cineole **66.1%**
alpha-pinene **14.7%**
3-methylbutanal **0.15%**
isoamyl isovalerate **0.02%**

Other significant constituents

limonene **3%**
aromadendrene **2.2%**
pinocarvone **1%**
alpha-terpinyl acetate **0.88%**
globulol **0.47%**
alpha-terpineol **0.44%**
beta-pinene **0.35%**
terpinen-4-ol **0.13%**

Eucalyptus oil is best known for its ability to help clear nasal or sinus congestion. It is used in small amounts to flavor lozenges and candy. Eucalyptus oil is used to add freshness to laundry detergents, especially for woolens and delicates. It is also a solvent for various adhesives.

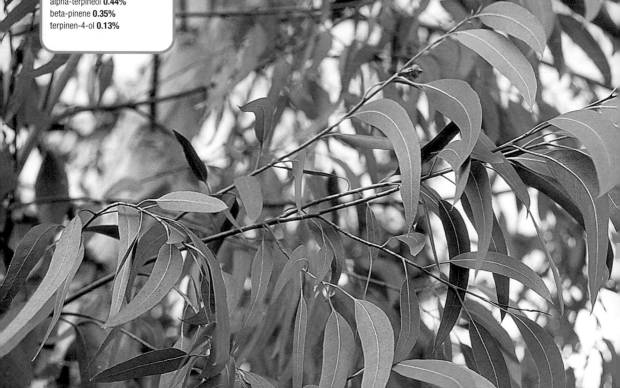

Traditional aromatherapy uses

Eucalyptus oil is traditionally used as a decongestant in respiratory infections, because it reputedly thins the mucous and acts as an expectorant, helping people cough up excess mucous. It is also used for aches and pains due to its rubefacient (warming) effects.

Ailments and remedies

Blocked sinuses and tight coughs Add 1 drop of Eucalyptus oil to a glass or ceramic bowl of hot tap water. Bend your head over the bowl and cover with a towel. Inhale the steam, either through your nose or your mouth, aiming to get as much Eucalyptus oil as possible onto your respiratory membranes. Blow your nose after 4 or 5 breaths, and repeat until you feel some relief from congestion.

Feverish aches and pains (e.g. influenza) Add 2 drops of Eucalyptus oil to 1 tablespoon of vegetable oil, and rub onto the affected joints and limbs. Put on old pajamas, and wrap yourself warmly to allow the Eucalyptus oil to penetrate your body. Reapply every couple of hours until the aches subside.

Why it works

1,8-cineole is also known as eucalyptole because it gives Eucalyptus oil its characteristic eucalyptus odor. Eucalyptus oil with major amounts of eucalyptole is used to help expel mucous in respiratory infections and for the relief of muscular aches and pains. Liniments often contain some proportion of Eucalyptus oil due to its warming effects on the skin.

Alpha-pinene adds to the warming effects of eucalyptole, and also contributes some antibacterial properties.

3-methylbutanal and **isoamyl isovalerate** have pungent odors that some people find unpleasant. They could also contribute to mucous membrane irritation during inhalation, which may have a beneficial effect if trying to cough up mucous.

Caution: Both 1,8-cineole and Eucalyptus oil are listed in the poisons schedule of most countries, and must be stored in poison bottles. Store all essential oils away from children, in the same way as any other medicine. Do not take Eucalyptus oil internally. As little as one tablespoon of Eucalyptus oil taken internally has had toxic effects on children.

Do not use Eucalyptus oil as an inhalation for babies under 12 months, or people who are prone to asthma, because 1,8-cineole can trigger constriction of the airways.

m vulgare var. *dulce*

Sweet Fennel

Fennel is used as a vegetable and a spice, although the essential oil is only extracted from the seeds. The seeds are found at the end of the spikes on the umbrella-shaped flowering parts from which the plant's family name Umbelliferae is taken. Cousins of Fennel—including Aniseed, Angelica, Cumin, Dill, and Yarrow—also produce aromatic essential oils in their seeds.

In India, sugar-coated seeds of Fennel and Aniseed are constituents of paan, the digestive and breath-freshening chewing mixture taken after a hot, pungent curry meal. Sweet Fennel tea has been used medicinally to help regulate menstrual periods, and to promote lactation, although there have not been sufficient scientific studies fully to determine the mode of action or the effective dosages. Fennel oil is produced by steam distillation of the seeds. The variety used in aromatherapy is known as Sweet Fennel.

Traditional aromatherapy uses

Fennel oil has been used to help relieve the cramping from menstrual pain, and to help regulate irregular menstrual cycles. Taken in the form of a tea, Fennel has been used to reduce intestinal spasms and flatulence. When massaged into the lower limbs and kidney

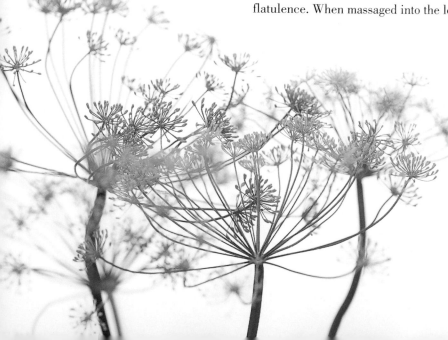

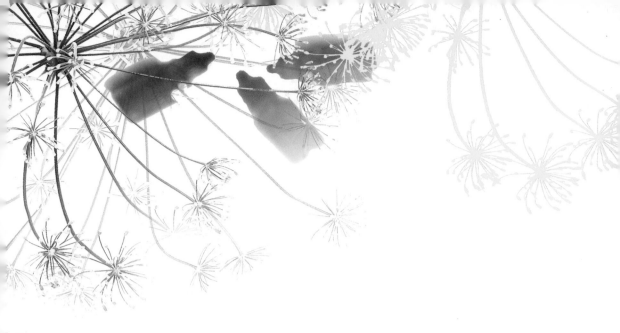

area the oil has a diuretic effect. As a result it is sometimes recommended for use in cellulitis and other sluggish circulation problems.

Ailments and remedies

Menstrual pain Add 5 drops of Fennel oil to a teaspoon of vegetable oil and apply in small circular stroking motions to the area above the uterus and lower back.

Bowel spasms and flatulence Apply the oil in the proportions as above, but massage the abdomen in a clockwise direction starting at the person's bottom right (see Basil oil, page 124).

Why it works

Anethole gives Sweet Fennel oil its strong aniseed-like aroma. So-called Bitter Fennel has a more pungent aroma and may contain compounds such as butanolide that give an unpleasant musky smell to the oil. Anethole may act as a mild estrogen, which supports Sweet Fennel oil's use as a menstrual regulator.

Methyl chavicol and **anethole** are antispasmodics acting on the aching muscles of internal organs. This would account for Sweet Fennel's effects on intestine, uterus, and possibly even bronchioles.

Sweet Fennel

Turkey

Active constituents

Trans-anethole **80%**
methyl chavicol **4.5%**

Other known constituents

limonene **6%**
fenchone **2%**
anisaldehyde **1%**
1,8-cineole **0.4%**
cis-anethole **0.3%**
carvone **0.1%**
octanal **0.1%**

Caution:

Do not use Sweet Fennel oil on people with liver disease, or babies under 12 months old as anethole can pose a challenge to the liver. In high doses anethole may affect estrogen-dependent cancers. However, the amounts absorbed during an abdominal massage or inhalation as described above are extremely unlikely to pose any risks. If concerned, avoid use of Sweet Fennel oil with endometriosis and breast and ovarian cancers.

Helichrysum italicum

Immortelle

The name for this fragrant Mediterranean plant (also known as the Curry Plant) comes from the length of time the flowers stay colorful. The golden yellow blooms are also referred to as "paper daisies." An alternative botanical name is *Helichrysum augustifolium*. It was used as a liver tonic, to relieve chronic respiratory conditions, and as a remedy for bruises and sprains. A related species indigenous to North America was said, by Native Americans, to be a cure for rattlesnake bite.

The odor of the oil is reminiscent of Roman Chamomile (*Anthemis nobilis*, see page 50), although it has its own distinctive character, which some people say reminds them of used teabags. The oil has a reputation for improving scars, and some sources suggest that it can prevent scarring if applied to the wound during healing. The oil is extracted from the flowering tops by steam distillation, but can also be extracted with solvents.

Traditional aromatherapy uses

Immortelle oil is best known for its anti-inflammatory and wound-healing effects. In chronic respiratory conditions, where there is ongoing inflammation, a steam inhalation with Immortelle oil can accelerate healing in the lungs and airways. In herbal medicine, it was used as an astringent and bitter liver tonic.

Ailments and remedies

Bruises and sprains Add 5 drops of Immortelle oil to 1 tablespoon of vegetable oil and rub gently into the bruise or sprain. Then use a cold pack or a bag of frozen peas as a cold compress, which will help to lessen the bloodflow to the area and reduce swelling. Rest with the compress on the sprain for up to 15 minutes, but not longer. If the tissue becomes too cold, it can have a negative effect on the healing process.

Chronic respiratory infections Add 2 drops of Immortelle oil to a bowl of boiling water and do a steam inhalation: Cover your head with a towel, and inhale through the mouth to coat the surfaces of the throat and lungs.

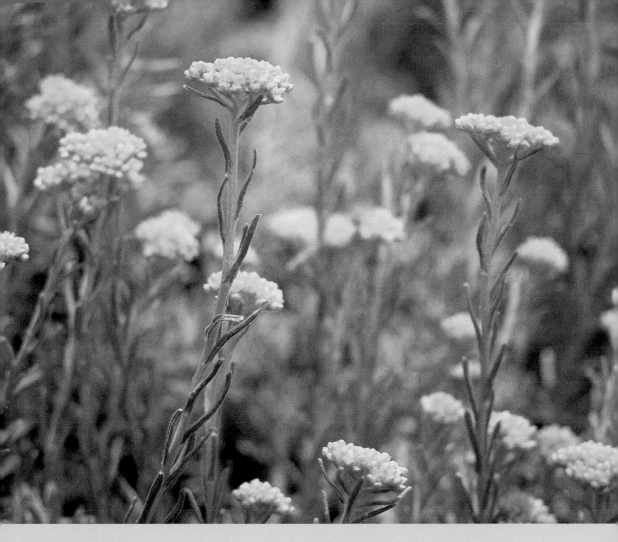

Why it works

Alpha-pinene gives the oil its mild antibacterial properties, and probably helps in the relief of respiratory conditions.

Gamma-curcumene and **alpha-curcumene** are compounds also found in Ginger oil (*Zingiber officinale*, see page 154). They have anti-inflammatory properties, and are thought to prevent the formation of stomach ulcers in rats.

Neryl acetate gives the oil a pleasant floral odor, and in some sources is recorded as high as 65%, which probably depends on the time of harvest and what proportion of leaf material was included in the distillation. In tests, it may contribute to relaxing and calming properties.

Beta-caryophyllene also has known anti-inflammatory properties, and may contribute to the relief of bruises and sprains.

Italidiones are thought to act as a clean-up tool for dead cells, helping bruises and sprains heal by removing dead matter. Certainly the oil has a reputation as a scar-improving oil, and some experts suggest that it can prevent scarring if applied to a wound while it is healing.

Immortelle

Active constituents

alpha-pinene **21.7%**
gamma-curcumene **10.4%**
italidiones **8%**
neryl acetate **6.1%**
beta-caryophyllene **5%**
alpha-curcumene **4%**

Other known constituents

beta-selinene **6%**
italicene **4%**
alpha selinene **3.6%**
isoitalicene **1.5%**
neryl propionate **1.2%**
2-methylbutyl angelate **0.6%**
nerolidol **0.3%**
borneol **0.2%**
italicene epoxide **0.2%**
italicene ethers **0.2%**

Jasminum grandiflorum
Jasmine

There are two species of Jasmine vine that are growncommercially for their essential oil: *Jasminum grandiflorum* and *J. sambac*. Both originated in India and Persia, but were brought to Spain and the rest of Europe by way of Africa and the Moorish invasions. The *sambac* oil is mainly produced in India, and the *grandiflorum* oil in North Africa and France.

In China, green tea is scented with jasmine flowers from *J. paniculatum*, and served as a digestive stimulant after oily meals, removing bad breath and soothing the nerves. The oil is obtained from the white star-shaped flowers by solvent extraction, which produces an extract. In India, Jasmine oil is mixed with Sandalwood oil, creating an attar of jasmine. This is used as a perfume and as an aid to meditation. Garlands of *J. sambac* flowers are offered to honored guests and as part of worship in the temple. In the world of perfumery, Jasmine is known as the "queen of flowers" for its intense floral note. The oil is very expensive, and one of the world's most costly perfumes, "Joy" by Jean Patou, has pure Jasmine oil among its ingredients.

Traditional aromatherapy uses

As Jasmine oils are so expensive, they are mainly used in aromatherapy for the treatment of mental and emotional conditions, in particular depression and difficulties associated with sexual response in both men and women. Some sources suggest that the oil is useful in childbirth, aiding contractions when rubbed on the abdomen, but it is important that the mother likes the smell of the oil and agrees to use it.

Ailments and remedies

Sensual enjoyment Run a deep, warm bath, turn out the lights, and light a candle. Before getting into the bath, anoint your throat and upper chest with 3 drops of Jasmine oil diluted in vegetable oil. Because Jasmine is so expensive, most stores carry a prediluted product.

Depressive moods Carry a small bottle of Jasmine oil with you, and sniff it whenever you feel the depression striking. The odor of Jasmine has been shown to be stimulating, so it will create a sense of alert well-being—provided you like the smell!

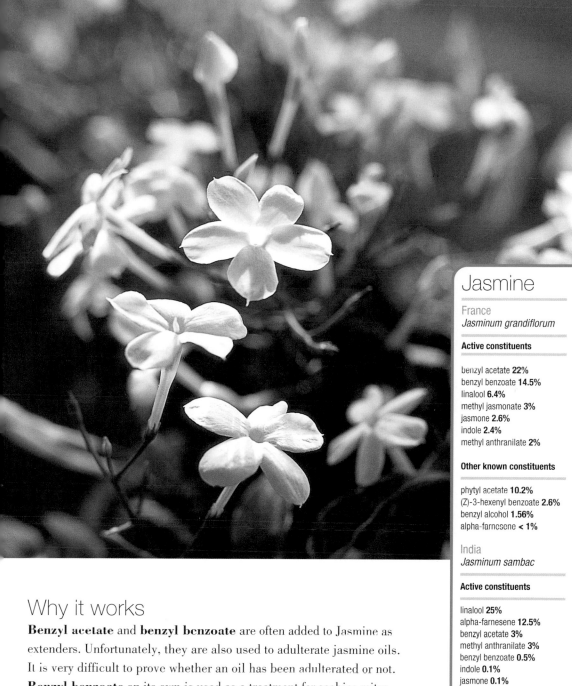

Jasmine

France
Jasminum grandiflorum

Active constituents

benzyl acetate **22%**
benzyl benzoate **14.5%**
linalool **6.4%**
methyl jasmonate **3%**
jasmone **2.6%**
indole **2.4%**
methyl anthranilate **2%**

Other known constituents

phytyl acetate **10.2%**
(Z)-3-hexenyl benzoate **2.6%**
benzyl alcohol **1.56%**
alpha-farnesene **< 1%**

India
Jasminum sambac

Active constituents

linalool **25%**
alpha-farnesene **12.5%**
benzyl acetate **3%**
methyl anthranilate **3%**
benzyl benzoate **0.5%**
indole **0.1%**
jasmone **0.1%**
methyl jasmonate **0.01%**

Other known constituents

(-)-germacra-1,6-dien-5-ol **20%**
phytol **8%**
(Z)-3-hexenyl benzoate **5%**
benzyl alcohol **3%**
p-cresol **0.05%**
eugenol **0.05%**

Why it works

Benzyl acetate and **benzyl benzoate** are often added to Jasmine as extenders. Unfortunately, they are also used to adulterate jasmine oils. It is very difficult to prove whether an oil has been adulterated or not.
Benzyl benzoate on its own is used as a treatment for scabies mites.
Linalool has sedative properties on the nervous system. *J. sambac* would therefore be expected to be more relaxing than *J. grandiflorum* oil.
Alpha-farnesene is present in higher quantities in *J. sambac* oil, and may give the oil greater anti-inflammatory properties, for example in the treatment of painfully engorged breasts.
Methyl jasmonate, jasmone, indole, and **methyl anthranilate** provide the intense characteristic jasmine odor and may be responsible for Jasmine oil's euphoric and stimulating effects.

Juniperus communis
Juniper

The dried ripe berries of Juniper bushes are used in cooking and as the flavor for gin. The berries are dark blue when ripe, and must be handpicked to avoid contamination with the green unripe berries that occur on the bush at the same time.

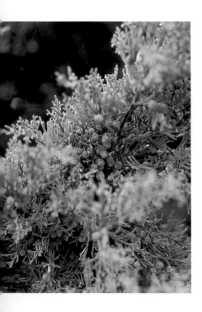

As with most trees of the Juniperus genus, *J. communis* produces a resin when the trunk is damaged, but this is not used commercially. Another species of Juniper, *J. oxycedrus* produces a resinous oil known as Cade oil. Cade oil, like coal tar, was used to treat eczema and dermatitis, but is not employed at present in aromatherapy. Juniper oil is steam distilled from the berries and has a characteristic odor that is not dissimilar from Pine oil (see page 132).

Juniper oil is traditionally considered to be a remedy for bladder problems, and for fluid retention, or "dropsy," caused by cardiac or liver malfunction. Some sources caution against the use of Juniper oil during pregnancy because of its supposed abortifacient effects. While it is likely that this caution derives from a confusion with *J. sabina*, which produces an oil known as Savin oil, it is advisable to avoid all Juniper oils during pregnancy. Savin oil showed toxic effects on rat embryos, causing early miscarriage.

Traditional aromatherapy uses

Juniper berry oil is used in aromatherapy for edematous conditions (swelling due to accumulation of fluids), particularly those relating to inflammatory conditions, such as rheumatism, gout, and arthritis. It is believed that the diuretic properties of the oil help purge the joints of toxins, although no research has conclusively proved this.

Ailments and remedies

Swollen joints Add 5 drops of Juniper berry oil to 1 tablespoon of vegetable oil, and massage into the affected joints. Repeat up to six times a day, and also drink more water (preferably filtered) to help the cleansing diuretic process.

Oily skin Add 1 drop of Juniper berry oil to a bowl of warm water and squeeze a facecloth into the mixture. Apply to the face, pressing the palms gently into the face. You can also do a mini face massage, though if there is acne present, this may be too painful. The Juniper will act as an astringent.

Why it works

Alpha-pinene provides the pine-like odor of Juniper oil, and also probably contributes to its diuretic properties. Alpha-pinene is a mild antiseptic and contributes to Juniper Berry oil's use for joint pain.

Beta-farnesene, **gamma-elemene**, and **beta-caryophyllene** have anti-inflammatory effects. Oil extracted from Juniper leaves and twigs has a major component of thujopsene which has not been scientifically tested.

> Caution: Juniper oil can deteriorate easily. It should be stored in the refrigerator, for a maximum of 12 months, and not used on the skin if it is old as it can cause irritation.
>
> Juniper oil is contraindicated for people with kidney problems and during pregnancy.

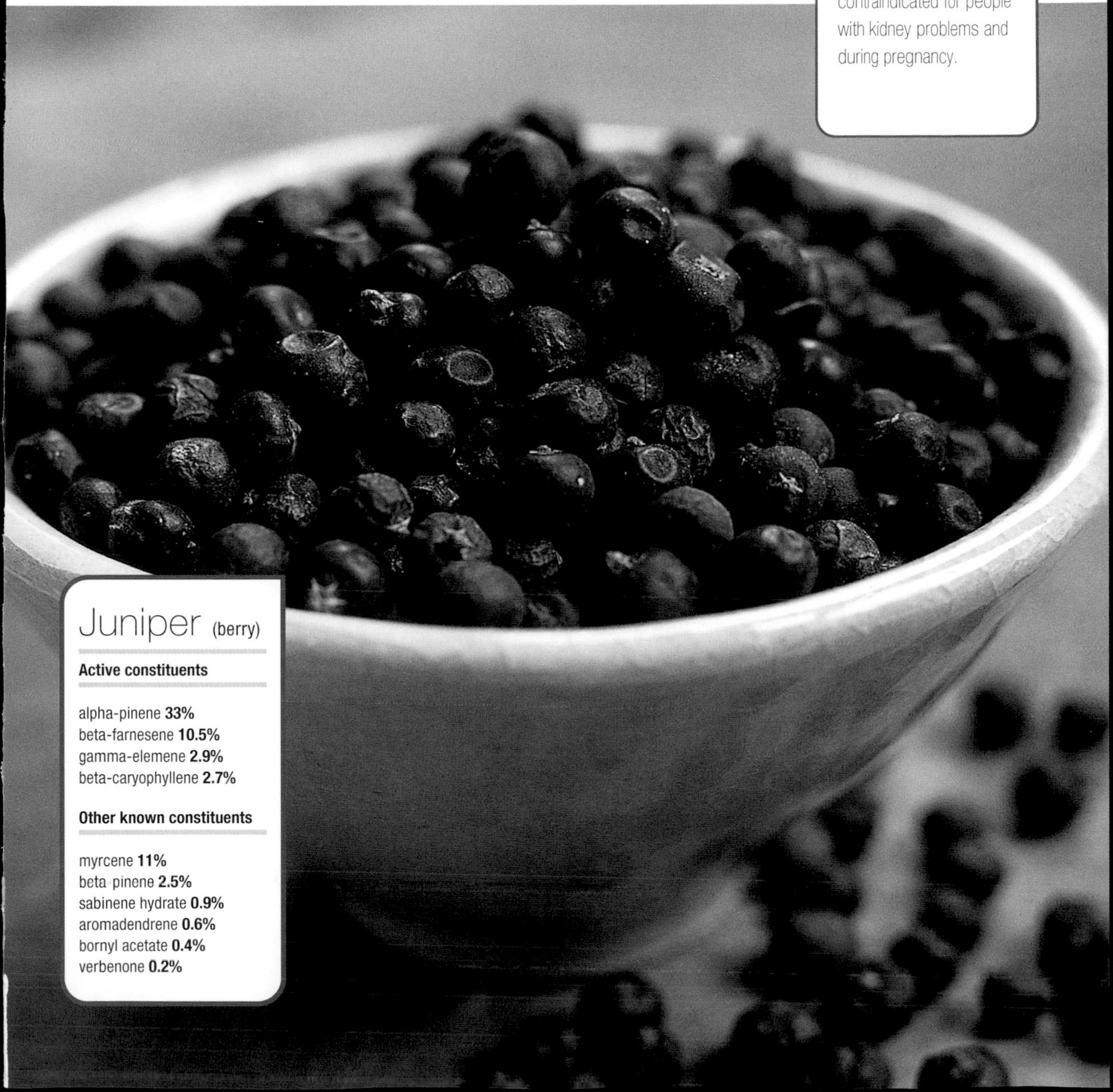

Juniper (berry)

Active constituents

alpha-pinene **33%**
beta-farnesene **10.5%**
gamma-elemene **2.9%**
beta-caryophyllene **2.7%**

Other known constituents

myrcene **11%**
beta-pinene **2.5%**
sabinene hydrate **0.9%**
aromadendrene **0.6%**
bornyl acetate **0.4%**
verbenone **0.2%**

Juniperus virginiana

Cedarwood, Virginia

The name Cedar is applied to many different species of trees, some from the Pinaceae family, which have the genus name *Cedrus*, others from the Cupressaceae family, with either *Cupressus* or *Juniperus* as their genus name. Cedar trees grow all around the world, the most famous being *Cedrus libani*, the Cedar of Lebanon referred to in biblical texts. The wood of these trees exudes a fragrant balsamic woody odor.

In the fragrance industry and in aromatherapy catalogs, the different Cedarwood oils are referred to by their place of origin; for example, Cedarwood Atlas (*Cedrus atlantica*) comes from the Atlas mountains of Morocco. The Virginian and Texas Cedarwood oils (*Juniperus mexicana*) were first identified in those states, but are now produced in North Carolina.

The thick, viscous Virginia Cedarwood oil is produced by steam distillation of shavings and chips of heartwood. The *Juniperus* oils are similar to one another in odor, and have a characteristic reddish-orange color. You can buy rectified oil, which is pale yellow, but this is not recommended for aromatherapy.

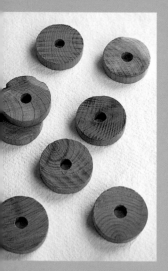

Cedarwood exudes a balsamic woody odor that repels moths, making it ideal for mothballs.

Traditional aromatherapy uses

The Atlas and Virginia Cedarwood oils are used to treat itching skin and bronchitis. They are also a component of various muscle rubs. The Virginia, Texas, and China Cedarwood oils are primarily used in perfumery for their strong woody scent.

Ailments and remedies

Itchy skin Add 5 drops of Virginia Cedarwood oil to 1 tablespoon of Sweet Almond vegetable oil and massage into the affected area. Repeat as often as needed to help assuage the itch.

Bronchitis Add 5 drops of Virginia Cedarwood to 1 teaspoon of vegetable oil and massage into the throat and upper chest just before going to sleep. This should help soothe the coughing during the night. You can also add 2 drops of Virginia Cedarwood to a bowl of hot water for a steam inhalation, breathing in through the mouth to coat the linings of the lungs.

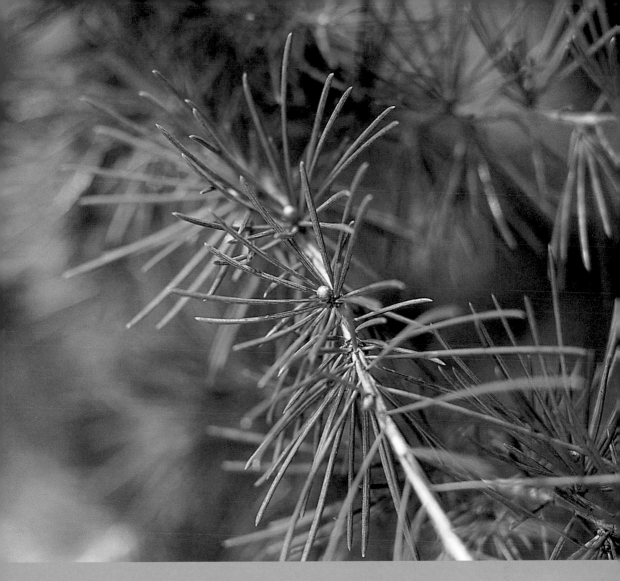

Why it works

Alpha-cedrene has been shown to have antibacterial properties in tests against organisms like *Candida albicans*, which causes thrush infections. It requires more research to determine whether it is effective against thrush in humans.

Thujopsene and **cedrol** have not been extensively analyzed for their individual therapeutic properties. However, from their chemical structure, they are all likely to possess anti-inflammatory properties, supporting the traditional uses of the oils.

Alpha-bisabolol is an example of a compound that has been shown to have anti-inflammatory properties. Alpha-bisabolol is one of the active components in German Chamomile oil (*Matricaria chamomilla*, see page 106), but it is probably not present in enough quantities in Cedarwood oil to have significant effect.

Cedarwood, Virginia

Active constituents

alpha-cedrene **21.1%**
thujopsene **21.3%**
cedrol **22.2%**
alpha-bisabolol **0.6%**

Other known constituents

Beta-cedrene **8.2%**
alpha-selinene **3.0%**
himachalene **2.1%**
widdrol **2.3%**
acoradiene, chamigrene,
curcumene, alaskene, cuparene
all **<1%** each

Laurus nobilis

Bay Laurel
{or Sweet Bay}

Bay Laurel trees are grown throughout the Mediterranean region and are noted for their glossy dark green leaves and black berries. The essential oil is derived from the dried leaves, which are also used in cooking. Bay leaves are a key component of bouquet garni, the bunch of herbs that is traditionally added to the stockpot.

The expression "to look to one's laurels" derives from the ancient Greek custom of honoring champions with a crown of bay laurel leaves. The berries also produce an essential oil and a vegetable oil, but neither of these is used in aromatherapy. Crushing the leaves yields the characteristic eucalyptus-like odor with an undertone of spicy clove.

Confusingly, there are several other species of tree that produce an essential oil known as Bay oil, but their botanic names are different, and so is the oil they produce. Most notable is the so-called West Indian Bay (*Pimenta racemosa*) and the closely related Allspice (*P. dioica*) from the Myrtaceae family. Both leaves and berries contain essential oils, which smell similar to Clove oil (*Eugenia caryophyllus*). These oils are used in the flavor industry, and are often ingredients in men's fragrances.

Traditional aromatherapy uses

Bay Laurel oil is used as an expectorant and decongestant (see Eucalyptus oil, page 88). Some sources also suggest that Bay Laurel oil can be used for headaches, especially sinus-related headaches. The oil is used as a digestive aid, stimulating the appetite and the production of salivary juices. Liniments and arthritis creams can contain Bay Laurel oil.

Ailments and remedies

Poor appetite Use three drops in a vaporizer while meals are being prepared. The spicy smell of the oil will awaken the salivary glands and set the stomach gurgling.

Stiff muscles or arthritis Take one tablespoon of vegetable oil and add 5 drops of Bay Laurel oil. Rub as vigorously as possible into the affected area, stimulating bloodflow with the friction of rubbing. A warm compress or heat pack can be applied afterward to aid the penetration of the oil and continue its warming action. However, some sources caution that there is a mild risk of irritation.

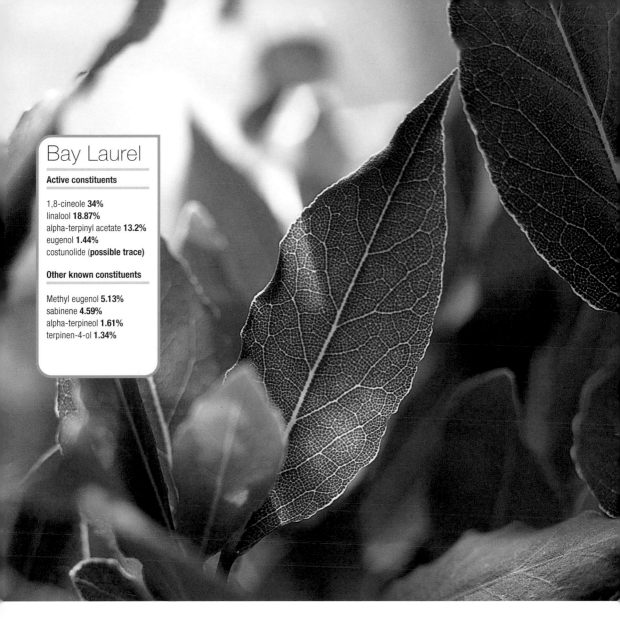

Bay Laurel

Active constituents

1,8-cineole **34%**
linalool **18.87%**
alpha-terpinyl acetate **13.2%**
eugenol **1.44%**
costunolide (**possible trace**)

Other known constituents

Methyl eugenol **5.13%**
sabinene **4.59%**
alpha-terpineol **1.61%**
terpinen-4-ol **1.34%**

Why it works

1,8-cineole is the main component of Bay Laurel oil, and is an expectorant and decongestant (see Eucalyptus oil [*Eucalyptus globulus*], page 88). 1,8-cineole also has warming properties and is used in liniments.

Eugenol content gives the oil a clove-like odor. It is responsible for the oil's antispasmodic and digestive properties. Eugenol also has mild anesthetic properties and is antibacterial.

Linalool contributes calming and sedative properties.

Alpha-terpinyl acetate contributes a pleasant lily-like note to the oil's odor.

Costunolide has been shown as a probable cause of skin allergies in people who handle bay laurel leaves. It should not be present in steam-distilled Bay Laurel oil above trace amounts.

Caution:

Eugenol can irritate skin and mucous membranes, so Bay Laurel oil smelling strongly of cloves should always be diluted in vegetable oil when using it on the skin. If you have other skin allergies, do not use Bay Laurel oil.

Lavandula angustifolia, L. officinale
Lavender

Lavender oil is one of the most popular oils in aromatherapy. Two species are used—the English lavender (*L. vera*) and the French lavender (*L. angustifolia*)—both of which yield a similar oil. French lavender grows wild all over southern Europe. The most highly prized lavender in aromatherapy is the so-called "wild crafted" Alpine French lavender, which is handpicked and distilled in small amounts by local farmers.

The oil is steam distilled from the flowering tops of lavender. The oil is clear and usually colorless, and has a sweet herbaceous smell characteristic of lavender. One of the problems for lavender growers is the cross-fertilization of different species of lavender to form hybrids. The odor of the oil varies markedly between the different species and hybrids (see Spike Lavender [*L. latifolia*], page 104). Lavender oil is more expensive than Spike Lavender oil, so sometimes unscrupulous producers blend the two to increase their profit margin. If the oil smells at all like Eucalyptus oil, it is probably such a blend.

Traditional aromatherapy uses

Lavender oil is traditionally seen as a first-aid kit in a bottle. It is useful to have on hand in the kitchen to apply to burns, and to take on picnics as a remedy for insect bites and stings. For those of an anxious disposition, it is supposed to have a relaxing effect, though some sources suggest that too much lavender has the opposite effect.

Ailments and remedies

Burns For sunburn and for little burns from spitting fat or from ironing, cover the burned area liberally in undiluted Lavender oil as quickly as possible. The oil will remove the sting and heat from the burn, and the skin should not blister. Reapply if any pain recurs.

Bites and stings Apply undiluted Lavender oil directly to the bite or sting. Reapply as needed until the swelling goes down and the pain diminishes.

Nervous insomnia and stress Use 3 drops in a vaporizer and vaporize in the bedroom for a half hour before going to sleep. Alternatively, put 1–2 drops on the pillow or near the neck of the pajamas, so that the odor can be inhaled. Another way is to add 3 drops to a warm bath and take the bath with lowered lights (a candle is good) just before going to bed.

Why it works

Linalool and **linalyl acetate** seem to have local analgesic and anesthetic effects.

Beta-caryophyllene, although only present in small amounts, would add to the anti-inflammatory effects of the oil.

Coumarins are present in trace amounts and can contribute to the sedative action of the oil. They may also help to lower blood pressure.

Terpinen-4-ol is an antibacterial agent, like linalool (see above). The two agents contribute effective anti-infectious properties.

Camphor and **1,8-cineole** are the two compounds that reduce the perfume value of Lavender oil. They also reverse the sedative and relaxing effects normally associated with the oil (compare Spike Lavender, *L. latifolia*, see page 104). The Lavender oil preferred by aromatherapists has minute amounts of camphor and 1,8-cineole, which combined in amounts greater than about 5% give the oil a eucalyptus-like odor.

Lavender
France

Active constituents

linalyl acetate **40%**
linalool **31.5%**
beta-caryophyllene **5.16%**
terpinen-4-ol **4%**
1,8-cineole **0.69%**
camphor **0.3%**
coumarins **(Trace)**

Other known constituents

(Z)-beta-ocimene **6.7%**
lavandulyl acetate **4.2%**
3-octanone **1.5%**
lavandulol **0.7%**

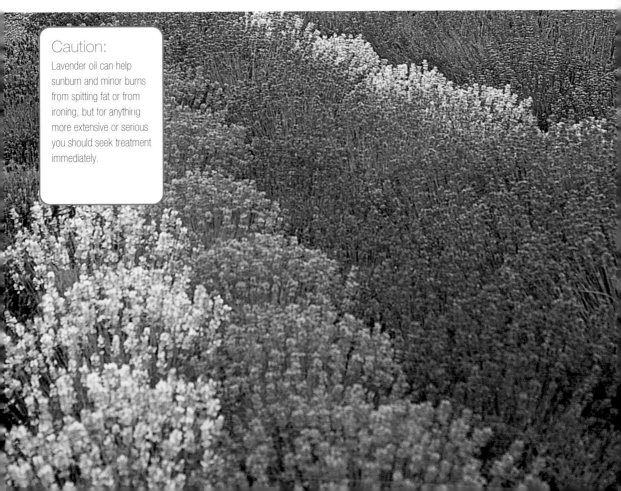

Caution:
Lavender oil can help sunburn and minor burns from spitting fat or from ironing, but for anything more extensive or serious you should seek treatment immediately.

Lavandula latifolia

Lavender, Spike

Spike Lavender, like Lavender (*L. angustifolia*, see page 102), is distilled from the flowering tops of the plants. It produces a higher yield of oil than Lavender, and is sometimes used to adulterate Lavender and Lavandin oils. Lavandin is a hybrid of Lavender, known as *L. hybrida* or *L. x intermedia*, and produces an oil in odor somewhere between Lavender and Spike Lavender.

The odor of Spike Lavender oil is similar to that of Lavender, but is also reminiscent of Rosemary oil. The odor of Lavandin oil is more lavender-like, but is somewhat coarser than that of Lavender oil, so it is mainly used in candle making, soaps, and detergents. There are various grades of Lavandin oil, such as "Super" and "Grosso," but for aromatherapy purposes, these grades are not especially relevant, all yielding oils that contain more camphor and cineole than *L. angustifolia*.

Traditional aromatherapy uses

Spike Lavender and Lavandin oils are not used extensively in aromatherapy, although there is no reason why they should not be, especially for respiratory infections. They may also provide relief for arthritic aches and pains, and poor circulation, because of their warming effects.

Ailments and remedies

Colds, influenza, bronchitis Add 3 drops of Spike Lavender to a bowl of boiling water and inhale the steam deeply into the lungs and sinuses. Cover the head with a towel to keep the vapors in, and continue the inhalation for 5–10 minutes. Repeat 3 times a day—and more, if possible.

Aches and pains Aches and pains in the joints, whether arthritic, sporting, or influenza-caused, can benefit from a rub with Spike Lavender oil. Add 5 drops of oil to 1 tablespoon of vegetable oil (or double the quantities), and rub onto the aching area. If you can tolerate it, rub vigorously, because this will also stimulate bloodflow to the area.

Why it works

1,8-cineole and **camphor** make Spike Lavender oil an excellent choice for colds, influenza, bronchitis, and sinusitis because they help to get rid of excess mucous. They also give Spike Lavender oil an odor reminiscent of

> Caution:
> Do not take Spike Lavender orally due to its 1,8-cineole and camphor content, which can cause toxic reactions in acute doses.

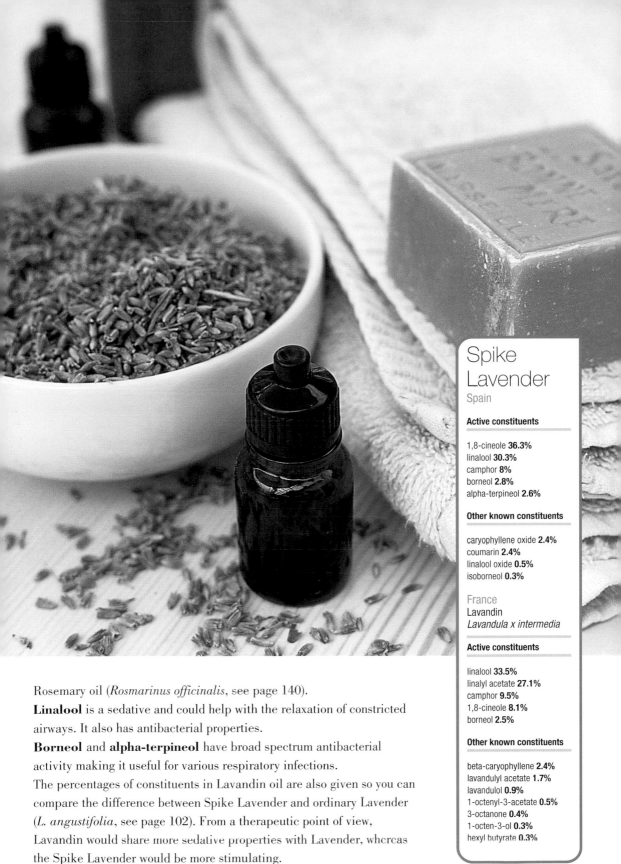

Spike Lavender
Spain

Active constituents

1,8-cineole **36.3%**
linalool **30.3%**
camphor **8%**
borneol **2.8%**
alpha-terpineol **2.6%**

Other known constituents

caryophyllene oxide **2.4%**
coumarin **2.4%**
linalool oxide **0.5%**
isoborneol **0.3%**

France
Lavandin
Lavandula x intermedia

Active constituents

linalool **33.5%**
linalyl acetate **27.1%**
camphor **9.5%**
1,8-cineole **8.1%**
borneol **2.5%**

Other known constituents

beta-caryophyllene **2.4%**
lavandulyl acetate **1.7%**
lavandulol **0.9%**
1-octenyl-3-acetate **0.5%**
3-octanone **0.4%**
1-octen-3-ol **0.3%**
hexyl butyrate **0.3%**

Rosemary oil (*Rosmarinus officinalis*, see page 140).

Linalool is a sedative and could help with the relaxation of constricted airways. It also has antibacterial properties.

Borneol and **alpha-terpineol** have broad spectrum antibacterial activity making it useful for various respiratory infections.

The percentages of constituents in Lavandin oil are also given so you can compare the difference between Spike Lavender and ordinary Lavender (*L. angustifolia*, see page 102). From a therapeutic point of view, Lavandin would share more sedative properties with Lavender, whereas the Spike Lavender would be more stimulating.

Matricaria chamomilla, M. recutita

Chamomile, German

There are several species of Chamomile, which are characterized by their white daisy-like flowers with yellow centers, and feathery leaves. The two types of Chamomile oil used in aromatherapy—German (*M. chamomilla*) and Roman chamomile (*Anthemis noblis*)—have very different chemical compositions and different therapeutic properties. Traditionally, the dried flowers of both chamomile species are used as herbal teas and decoctions.

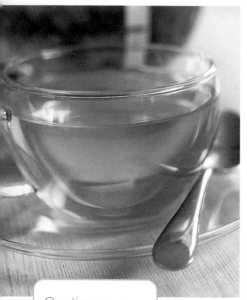

The tea is claimed to be soothing and sedative, and is often used for the treatment of children's digestive complaints. Most producers of Chamomile tea do not put the botanic name on the package, but the majority almost certainly use the English or Roman Chamomile, which has a sweet apple-like odor. German Chamomile flowers have a distinctive earthy smell, and supposedly produce a more bitter tea than the flowers of Roman Chamomile. The oil of German Chamomile is produced by steam distillation or CO_2 extraction of the flowers.

Traditional aromatherapy uses

German Chamomile oil is used for inflammatory and itchy conditions, and is also applied externally for the soothing of digestive problems. It has been used as a component of wound-healing blends.

Ailments and remedies

Itchy skin conditions Add 3 drops of German Chamomile to 1 teaspoon of vegetable oil or, if you have purchased the prediluted oil (usually 3% in Jojoba vegetable oil), use 1 teaspoon of that without additional dilution. Massage gently into the itchy area, and reapply as needed until soothed.

Insect bites and stings This is a first-aid situation, and the most effective use of the oil is to apply 1 or 2 drops undiluted directly to the bite or sting for rapid soothing.

Caution: People allergic to daisy-type flowers should test German Chamomile oil on normal skin before using it on inflamed areas. If the oil causes an irritation, wipe off immediately, then rinse the area with running cold water.

Sore eyes Make a cup of herbal Chamomile tea with 2 teabags. When the teabags are cool, place them on your closed eyelids and relax.

Why it works

Farnesene, alpha-bisabolol oxide A and B, and **alpha-bisabolol** all contribute to the anti-inflammatory properties of the oil.
Alpha-bisabolol has also been shown to speed up wound healing.
Chamazulene gives the steam-distilled oil its dark blue color, and contributes to its anti-inflammatory properties. The CO_2 extract is a pale yellow color as chamazulene is produced during the steam-distillation process.

German Chamomile

Active constituents

farnesene **27%**
chamazulene **17%**
alpha-bisabolol oxide B **11%**
alpha-bisabolol **9.5%**
alpha-bisabolol oxide A **8%**,

Other known constituents

Delta-cadinene **5.2%**
alpha-muurolene **3.4**
en-yn-dicycloether **0.7%**
beta-caryophyllene **0.5%**

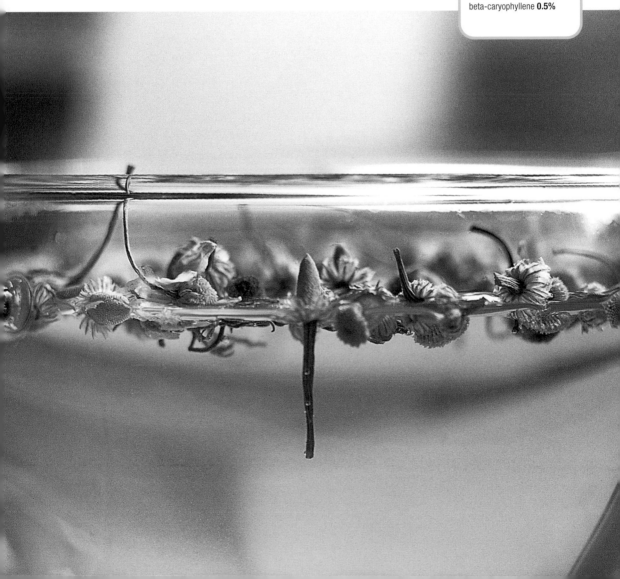

Melaleuca alternifolia

Tea Tree {Australian}

The name Tea Tree is given to a large number of swamp-growing shrubs and trees from the Myrtaceae family, growing in Australia and New Zealand. The name comes from the fact that the trees grow in or near water that is usually a clear brown tea color due to the tannins from the leaves and twigs that fall into it. Commercial growers now clone seedlings to ensure high oil quality. Melaleuca trees are also known as "paperbark" trees, because of their papery bark.

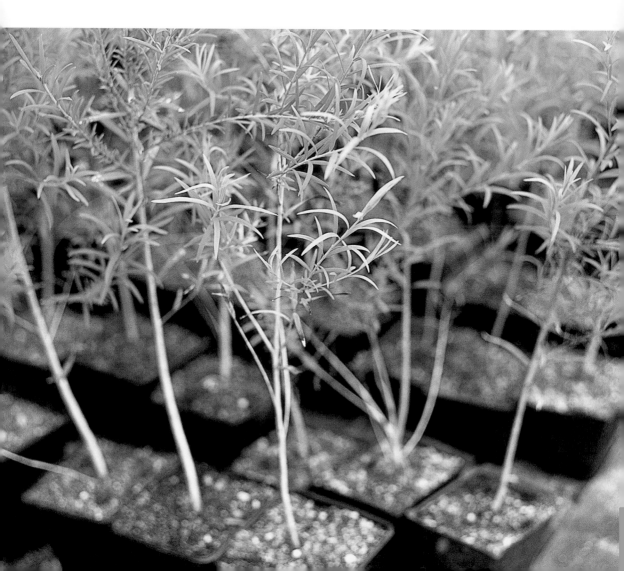

The oil is extracted from the leaves, and should be a clear, colorless to pale yellow liquid with a fresh medicinal odor. The darker the yellow, the more likely the oil is either old or oxidized. A yellow oil can still be used, but is likely to be more irritating.

Traditional aromatherapy uses

Tea Tree oil is primarily noted for its broad-spectrum antibacterial and antifungal effects, and recent research shows that it exhibits anti-inflammatory properties. It has been used in treatment of acne, boils, candida infections, tinea, sore throats, and other inflammatory infections. The aroma is not particularly valued, but can be blended with oils such as Lemongrass (*Cymbopogon citratus*, see page 82), or even Lemon Tea Tree (*Leptospermum petersonii*), to improve the odor.

Ailments and remedies

Genital candidiasis or thrush Add 3 drops of Tea Tree oil to a shallow bath, just before getting in. Dry yourself with a clean towel, and apply 3 drops of Tea Tree oil diluted in 1 teaspoon of vegetable oil. Reapply the oil blend throughout the day whenever the area is itchy. If you feel that the Tea Tree oil is not working at this concentration, increase the number of drops per teaspoon of vegetable oil by one drop per day, as long as it does not cause additional irritation.

To help the cure, avoid all sugar, alcohol, dairy, and processed starch foods for a period of 3 weeks while you are using the Tea Tree oil.

Respiratory Infections Add 3 drops of Tea Tree oil to a bowl of hot tap water and inhale the vapors with the head covered by a towel. Repeat 3–4 times per day until the infection is cleared.

Why it works

Terpinen-4-ol has antibacterial and antifungal properties. Both terpinen-4-ol and alpha-terpineol have been shown to have pain-relieving properties when applied topically to the skin.

Gamma-terpinene and **alpha-terpineol** also have antibacterial activity, and contribute to the oil's effectiveness against different types of infections.

1,8-cineole is a useful expectorant, but is considered a potential irritant.

Para-cymene is a known skin irritant. The level of para-cymene increases as the oil deteriorates over time, and also increases the yellow color and pungent resinous odor of the oil.

Tea Tree

Active constituents

terpinen-4-ol **45.4%**
gamma-terpinene **15.7%**
para-cymene **6.2%**
alpha-terpineol **5.3%**
1,8-cineole **3%**

Other known constituents

alpha-terpinene **7.1%**
alpha-pinene **2.1%**
limonene **1.4%**

Caution: To avoid risk of skin irritation, always dilute Tea Tree oil in vegetable oil. Do not use old or yellow-colored Tea Tree oil on the skin.

Avoid taking Tea Tree oil internally, as it can cause oral toxicity.

Melaleuca leucadendron
Cajuput

Cajuput (or Cajeput) oil is produced from the leaves and twigs of the Swamp Paperbark (a name shared by several other *Melaleuca* species, its alternative botanical name is *M. cajuputii*). The paperbark trees of Australia and Southeast Asia grow in swampy areas, and many produce essential oils of one kind or another, although the *M. leucadendron* (Cajuput), *M. alternifolia* (Tea Tree), and *M. quinquinervia* (Niaouli) oils are the most available at this stage.

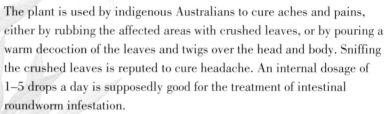

The plant is used by indigenous Australians to cure aches and pains, either by rubbing the affected areas with crushed leaves, or by pouring a warm decoction of the leaves and twigs over the head and body. Sniffing the crushed leaves is reputed to cure headache. An internal dosage of 1–5 drops a day is supposedly good for the treatment of intestinal roundworm infestation.

The oil is steam distilled from the leaves of the tree, and should be a clear, colorless to pale yellow liquid, reminiscent of Eucalyptus oil.

Traditional aromatherapy uses

Cajuput oil is used in the following ways as an expectorant and sudorific in colds and flu. Both the expectorant (mucous-releasing) and the sudorific (sweat-inducing) properties are probably due to the 1,8-cineole. It is also used as a component of a liniment for muscular aches and pains. The anti-inflammatory properties of the sesquiterpenols, coupled with the rubefacient (warming) properties of the 1,8-cineole and para-cymene, are probably responsible for this use of the oil.

Ailments and remedies

Coughs, colds, and influenza Add 1–2 drops to a bowl of hot water and inhale the vapors, covering the head with a towel to keep the vapors concentrated around the head. Inhale through the nose and out through the mouth for sinus congestion, and inhale through the mouth and out through the nose for a chest infection.

Arthritis or muscular strain Add 5 drops of Cajuput oil to 1 tablespoon of vegetable oil and massage the affected area as firmly as is comfortable. If

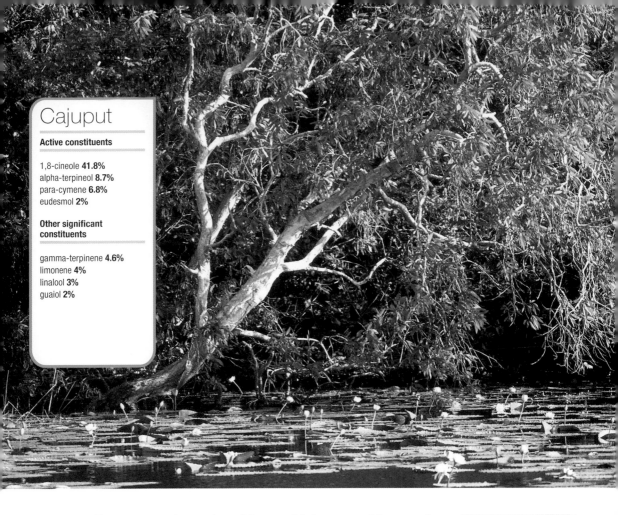

Cajuput

Active constituents

1,8-cineole **41.8%**
alpha-terpineol **8.7%**
para-cymene **6.8%**
eudesmol **2%**

Other significant constituents

gamma-terpinene **4.6%**
limonene **4%**
linalool **3%**
guaiol **2%**

there is no effect, increase the number of drops to 20 drops per tablespoon of vegetable oil and reapply. Cajuput oil will sting sensitive tissues, so avoid mucous membrane areas.

Why it works

Cajuput oil's high percentage of **1,8-cineole** makes it a good substitute for Eucalyptus oil (*Eucalyptus globulus*, see page 88) when treating respiratory infections.

Alpha-terpineol is a proven antibacterial and analgesic compound, adding to the usefulness of the oil in treating tight, painful coughs.

Eudesmol has been shown to alleviate the severity of experimentally induced seizures in animals. It would be interesting to find out whether Cajuput oil could be used in the prevention of epileptic seizures, though the percentage of eudesmol in the oil is probably too low to make much difference at the dosages used in aromatherapy.

The presence of **para-cymene** in Cajuput oil can cause skin irritation, though this irritation can be experienced as increasing warmth. Para-cymene probably contributes to Cajuput oil's usefulness for muscular aches and pains, along with 1,8-cineole.

Caution: Do not use Cajuput oil as an inhalation for babies under 12 months, or people who are prone to asthma as 1,8-cineole can trigger constriction of the airways.

Do not take Cajuput oil internally because 1,8-cineole can cause toxic effects.

To avoid risk of skin irritation, always dilute with vegetable oil.

Do not use Cajuput oil that has been exposed to the air as it may be oxidized. This can cause skin irritation.

Melaleuca quinquinervia
Niaouli

Niaouli oil is produced from the leaves and twigs of the *M. quinquinervia* paperbark tree, also known as *M. viridiflora*. It occurs in New Caledonia and Australia, and is used by Australian Aboriginals to cure aches and pains. Sniffing the crushed leaves is reputed to cure headaches. The oil can be used as a substitute for Eucalyptus oil or Cajuput oil in treating respiratory infections.

Niaouli
Madagscar

Active constituents

1,8-cineole **41.8%**
viridiflorol **18.1%**
alpha-terpineol **5%**

Other known constituents

limonene **5.5%**
beta-caryophyllene **5%**
alpha-pinene **5%**
ledol **2.5%**
caryophyllene oxide **0.6%**
(E)-nerolidol **0.4%**

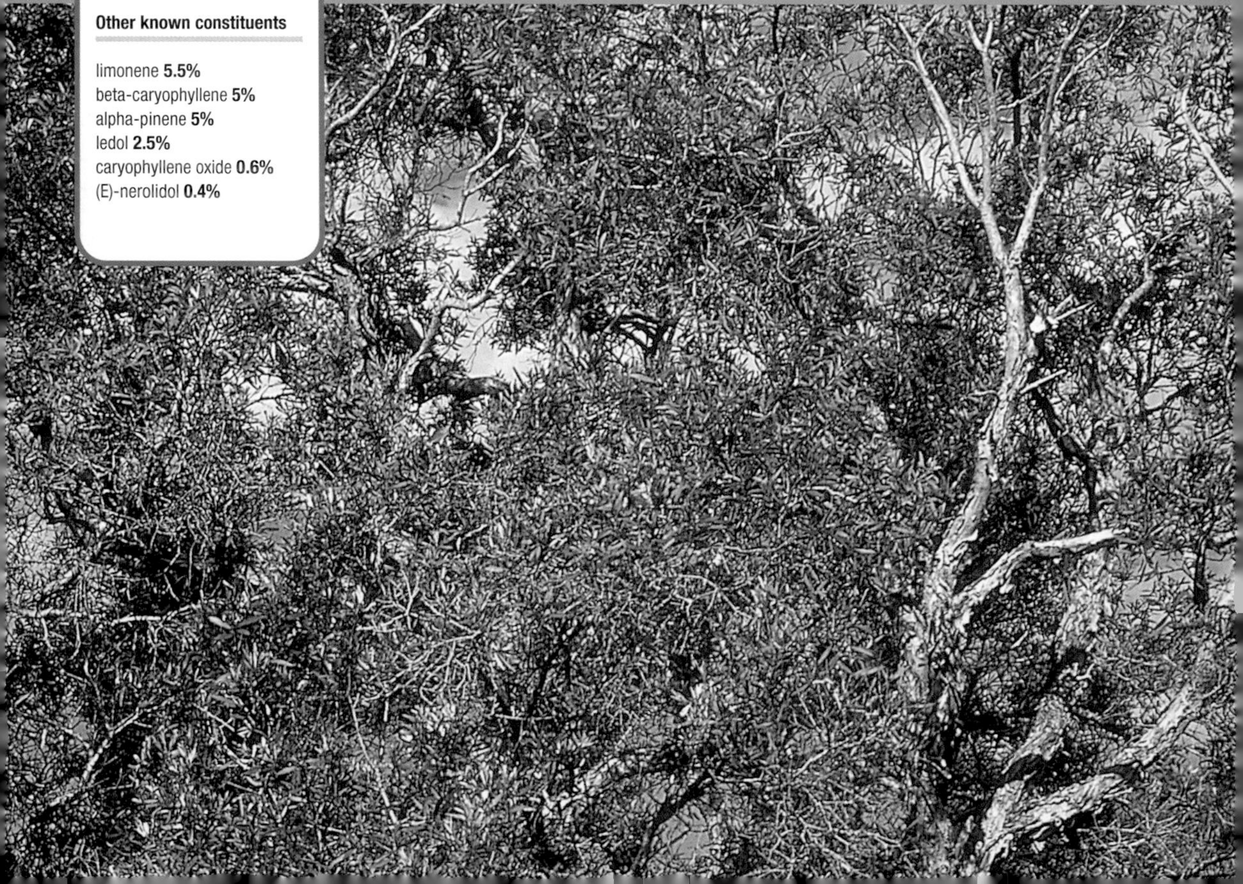

The pale yellowish oil is steam distilled and has a sweeter smell than Tea Tree oil (*M. alternifolia*, see page 108), somewhat similar to Eucalyptus (*Eucalpytus globulus*, see page 88). There is some suggestion that Niaouli oil is antiviral for viruses such as *Herpes simplex*, and that it has potential as an oral antimalarial agent, but this needs to be verified scientifically.

Traditional aromatherapy uses

Niaouli is used primarily for respiratory infections, in a similar way to Cajuput (*M. leucadendron*, see page 110) and Eucalyptus oil (*E. globulus*, see page 88). Some sources suggest it is useful in the treatment of varicose veins by helping to tone up the vein walls, but it is preferable to avoid massaging varicose veins. Niaouli can also be effective in alleviating muscular aches and pains.

Ailments and remedies

Bronchitis and viral colds Add 1 drop of Niaouli oil to a bowl of hot tap water, cover the head with a towel, and inhale the vaporizing oil through the nose and then through the mouth to coat the inside of the throat and nose. Repeat up to four times a day. Vaporize 3 drops of the oil in the bedroom before sleep to help prevent congestion during the night.

Muscular aches and pains Add 10 drops of Niaouli oil to 1 tablespoon of vegetable oil, and massage into the aching area, using gentle circular strokes. If possible, put a warm towel or compress over the affected part after the massage, to help bring blood to the area.

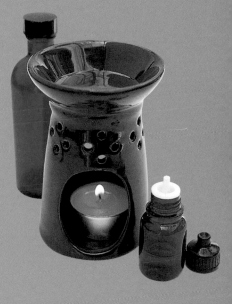

Why it works

There are two distinct types of oil produced by *M. quinquinervia*. Niaouli is the most common, and has a major percentage of 1,8-cineole. The other type is only recently available under the name Nerolina, which has a very different odor and proportion of chemicals. Nerolina oil has not been used in aromatherapy for very long, so we are unsure of its therapeutic effects at present.

1,8-cineole makes Niaouli oil useful for coughs and colds, helping cough up excess mucous. Niaouli oil can be used instead of Cajuput (*M. leucadendron*, see page 110) or Eucalyptus (*E. globulus*, see page 88) oil. Because the percentage of 1,8-cineole is lower in Niaouli oil than Eucalyptus, it is more suitable for young children and frail elderly people.

Viridiflorol may have anti-inflammatory properties, and is suggested by some sources to be useful as a vein tonic.

Alpha-terpineol has antibacterial and analgesic properties.

Caution: Do not use Niaouli oil as an inhalation for babies under 12 months, or people who are prone to asthma as 1,8-cineole can trigger constriction of the airways.

Do not use more than 1 or 2 drops in a steam inhalation, because the vapors can irritate the eyes if greater quantities are used.

Do not take Niaouli oil internally as 1,8-cineole can cause toxic effects.

Melissa officinalis

Melissa {or Lemon Balm}

Melissa comes from the Lamiaceae family of plants, along with the majority of essential oil-producing Mediterranean herbs, such as Peppermint, Rosemary, Sage, Lavender, Basil, Thyme, and Oregano. Its other name is Lemon Balm, which derives from its odor and the use of a decoction of its leaves to reduce stress and induce calm.

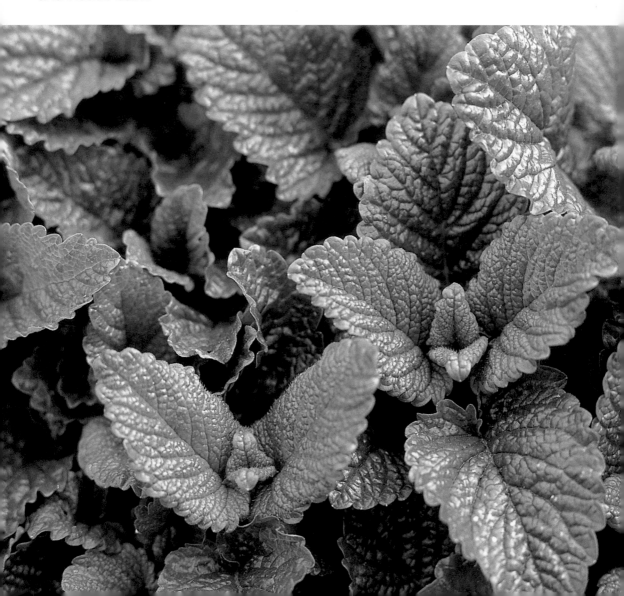

The oil is present in the plant in tiny amounts, so it is expensive to produce in commercial quantities. It is normally steam distilled, which yields a pale yellow oil with a characteristic lemony but also herbaceous scent. It is also available as a solvent-extracted product, but the therapeutic properties of the solvent extract have not been properly compared with those of the steam-distilled oil. (See Lemongrass, *Cymbopogon citratus*, page 82.)

Traditional aromatherapy uses

Melissa is traditionally used for its antispasmodic and calming effects. It is also used for its antiviral effects, particularly for viral infections such as cold sores.

Ailments and remedies

Nervous exhaustion Run a deep warm bath, and take the phone off the hook. Add 2 drops of Melissa oil to 1 teaspoon of vegetable oil and massage it into the chest, neck, and throat. Relax in the tub for 10–15 minutes with your eyes closed (but don't fall asleep!). Allow the aroma of the oil to relax you deeply. Melissa oil can be blended with 1 drop of Lavender oil, if you prefer.

Cold sores Use a clean cotton swab to dab a little undiluted Melissa oil onto the cold sore. Repeat hourly, if possible. The remedy works best if you can do it the moment you feel the first tingle, and before the blisters develop. You can still use it on the blisters, but it may sting. Be careful to dispose of the applicators in the garbage, so that no one else can become infected.

Why it works

Geranial, **neral**, and **citronellal** give Melissa oil its lemony odor. Percentages of these constituents vary. The oil is often adulterated with Lemongrass oil (*C. citratus*, see page 82) or Citronella oil (*C. winterianus*, see page 86), and sold as "reconstituted" Melissa oil. The combination of geranial and neral is commercially known as "citral."

Citral is an antifungal agent for conditions like tinea, and also repels insects. Citral can be irritating to the skin, especially if the oil is old.

> Caution: Do not use Melissa oil if you have sensitive skin as the citral content may cause irritation. If it does, wipe off the oil, and rinse the area with cold running water.

It is not yet clear which chemical components give Melissa oil its antispasmodic and calming effects. However, it is not citral, otherwise Lemongrass oil would also be considered antispasmodic and as a relaxant.

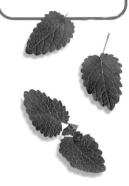

Melissa

Sardinia

Active constituents

geranial **40.62%**
neral **28.14%**
citronellal **6.48%**

Other known constituents

beta-caryophyllene **5.6%**
piperitone **2.3%**
alpha-muurolene **2.1%**
geraniol **2.0%**
6-methyl-5-hepten-2-one **0.07%**
3-octanone **0.09%**
linalool **0.3%**
geranyl acetate **0.09%**
germacrene-D **0.09%**

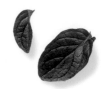

Mentha piperita
Peppermint

Peppermint is a hybrid of two mint species, *Mentha aquatica* and *M. spicata*, so it is more accurately written as *M. x piperita*, but most essential-oil suppliers use the name *M. piperita*. Peppermint is cultivated worldwide for its menthol content. Peppermint herbal tea has been used for centuries as an aid for indigestion, helping to soothe intestinal cramps.

The clear colorless oil is extracted from the aerial parts of the plant, mainly the leaves, and is usually harvested before flowering to prevent the inclusion of certain unpleasant-smelling molecules that are made by the plant after it flowers.

Traditional aromatherapy uses

Peppermint oil is used for cramping indigestion and nausea, and also for headaches and the relief of sinus pain. The cooling effect of Peppermint is felt by some people to be an irritation, or even a heating effect, depending on the dosage.

Ailments and remedies

Indigestion and intestinal cramps Add 1 drop of Peppermint oil to 1 teaspoon of vegetable oil and gently massage the abdomen in a clockwise direction, following the direction of the large intestine or colon.

Headache For a sinus headache, inhale the oil directly from the bottle, or add 1 drop to a tissue and inhale from that. Alternatively, add 1 drop of Peppermint oil to 1 teaspoon of vegetable oil and massage into the temples and brow, wherever the pain is worst. For a neck-related headache, massage the same dilution of oil into the seventh cervical vertebra at the base of the neck. You could add 1–2 drops of Lavender oil to the blend, especially if the headache is stress-related.

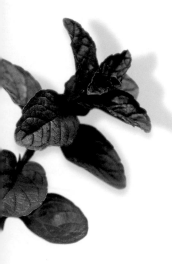

Caution:

Do not use Peppermint oil undiluted on the skin because it can cause a burning sensation in some people. It can also cause irritation to mucous membranes.

It is not recommended to use Peppermint oil with babies under 12 months, as the odor is so strong.

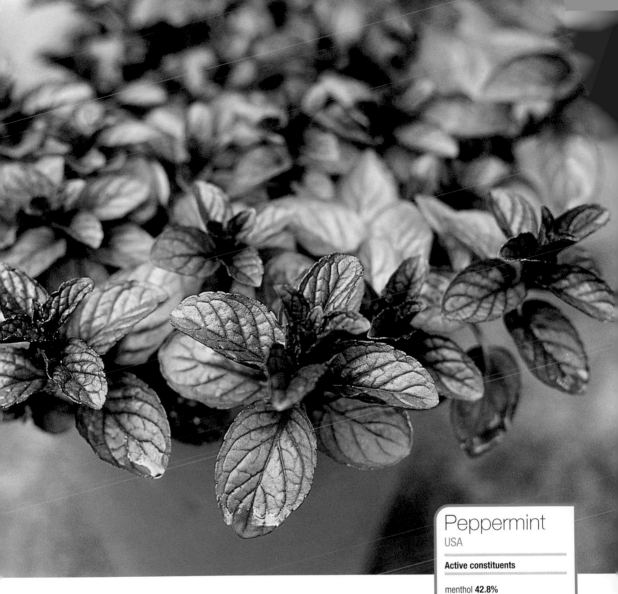

Why it works

Menthol, the major constituent of Peppermint oil, has been shown in tests to prevent the contraction of intestinal smooth muscle, and is considered to be the ingredient that makes Peppermint oil good for indigestion and intestinal cramping. Menthol also temporarily interacts with cold-sensitive nerve endings, causing a cooling sensation at the site of application. It is used in inhalation blends to help ease breathing in respiratory infections, as it increases the sensation of air in the sinuses and bronchioles. This effect could also help alleviate sinus headaches.

Menthone has a more penetrating odor than menthol and probably contributes to the alerting effect of the odor of Peppermint oil.

1,8-cineole adds to the respiratory clearing effect of menthol.

Peppermint
USA

Active constituents

menthol **42.8%**
menthone **19.4%**
1,8-cineole **5.2%**

Other known constituents

sabinene hydrate **6.6%**
neomenthol **4.2%**
isomenthone **3.2%**
beta-caryophyllene **2.3%**
menthofuran **2%**
limonene **1.6%**
pulegone **0.9%**

Mentha spicata

Spearmint

Spearmint oil is closely related to Peppermint (*Mentha piperita*), from the mint family. Both oils have been used for centuries to provide relief for indigestion. The essential oil of Spearmint is largely used in flavorings, and is commonly found in toothpastes, mouthwashes, confectionery, and chewing gum.

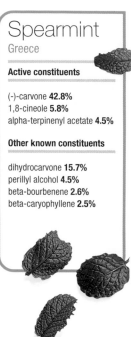

Spearmint
Greece

Active constituents

(-)-carvone **42.8%**
1,8-cineole **5.8%**
alpha-terpinenyl acetate **4.5%**

Other known constituents

dihydrocarvone **15.7%**
perillyl alcohol **4.5%**
beta-bourbenene **2.6%**
beta-caryophyllene **2.5%**

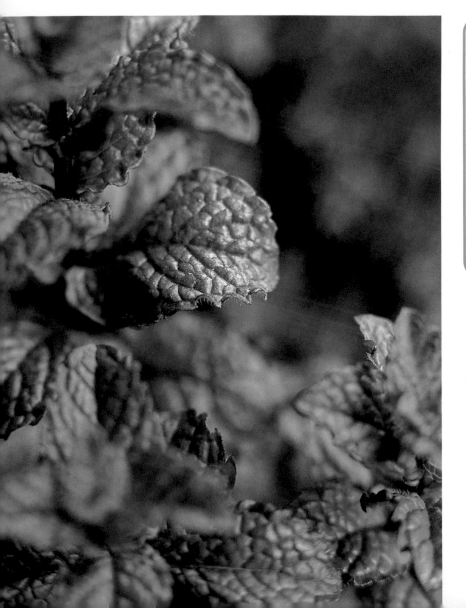

The oil is steam distilled from the leaves and stems of the plant, and is a clear, pale yellowish color. The two herbs can be distinguished by the different ways in which the leaves attach to the stems. Spearmint leaves appear to emerge directly from the stems, whereas Peppermint leaves have little stalks attaching them to the stems. Spearmint oil is sometimes confused with Caraway oil (*Carum carvi*), because they have similar odors, but Caraway oil is little used in aromatherapy.

Traditional aromatherapy uses

Spearmint oil is traditionally used for its antispasmodic effect on the smooth muscle of the gut, in a similar way to Peppermint oil. It is less pungent in odor than Peppermint oil, and some sources suggest that it is safer for use with colicky babies. It is also used for nausea and travel sickness, but this application depends on individual preference.

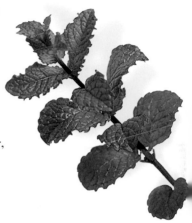

Ailments and remedies

Indigestion and colic Add 1 drop of Spearmint oil to a cup of warm water, and sip over a period of 5 minutes. For babies over 3 months old, give only 1 teaspoon of this mixture at a time, waiting for about 30 minutes before repeating the dose. Do not give more than 3 teaspoons of the spearmint flavored water per day. For breastfed babies under 3 months old, there is probably sufficient oil in the mother's milk if the mother drinks the remedy up to 3 times a day.

Nausea and travel sickness Put 1 drop of Spearmint oil on a tissue and inhale the aroma when the nausea strikes. If preferred, also drink the above indigestion remedy, or drink Spearmint herbal tea.

Why it works

Spearmint oil contains almost no menthol or menthone, which distinguishes it from Peppermint (*Mentha piperita*, see page 116).

Carvone has not been studied as intensively as menthol and menthone, but it is thought to have antispasmodic effects on the intestinal muscles, thus relieving indigestion. It also gives Spearmint oil its distinctive flavor and odor.

1,8-cineole is thought to help relieve respiratory congestion in coughs, colds, and sinusitis.

Alpha-terpinenyl acetate gives the odor of Spearmint oil a sweet floral note, and may be useful in helping with relaxation.

> Caution: It is not recommended to use essential oils for nausea caused by chemotherapy, as the odor can become linked with the experience of the nausea, and subsequently generate feelings of nausea when you later smell the same oil.
>
> As with Peppermint oil, Spearmint oil can cause irritation to the mucous membranes.

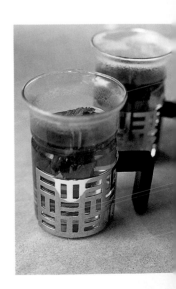

Myristica fragrans
Nutmeg

Nutmeg is an evergreen tropical tree, which produces a fleshy fruit and a hard seed that contains both a fatty oil and an essential oil. The scarlet fruit is dried and sold as mace, and powdered mace was originally used as a deterrent for vicious dogs, because it irritates the animal's eyes and nose. The seed is sold as a spice, either whole or powdered.

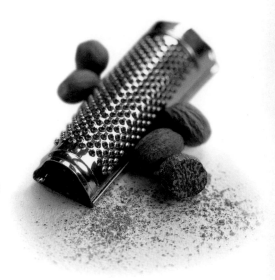

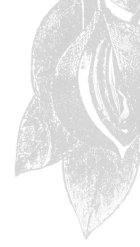

The name nutmeg comes from the old French *nois muguede*, which means "nut musk." In Victorian England, nutmeg powder was used as a flavoring for milk puddings and custards, especially for convalescents. It was reputed to be a tonic and gentle stimulant to help people get back on their feet. It was also used as a digestive tonic, and supposedly alleviated flatulence.

The essential oil is extracted from the dried nut by steam distillation, and is a clear pale yellow, with a spicy, penetrating odor similar that of Juniper berry oil (*Juniperus communis*, see page 96).

Traditional aromatherapy uses

Nutmeg oil is used in aromatherapy for its uplifting effects, particularly in cases of stress. It can also be used as a component in a liniment for muscular aches and pains and arthritis.

Ailments and remedies

Stress-related depressive moods Add 3 drops of Nutmeg oil and 3 drops of Mandarin oil to a vaporizer to boost low mood states. You can also take a small bottle of Nutmeg oil and inhale the aroma from time to time through the day to help maintain a happier state.

Muscular aches and pains Add 5 drops of Nutmeg oil to 1 tablespoon of vegetable oil and apply to the affected area. A heat pack will help bring blood to the area and reduce the stiffness.

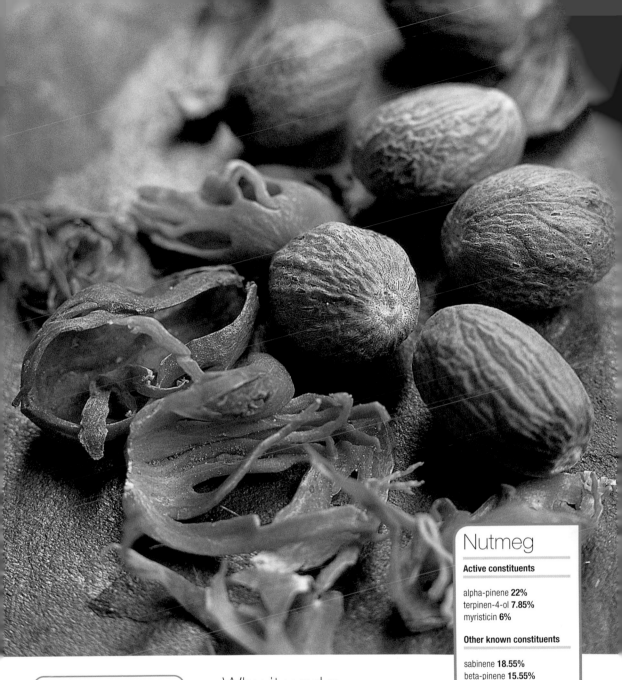

Nutmeg

Active constituents

alpha-pinene **22%**
terpinen-4-ol **7.85%**
myristicin **6%**

Other known constituents

sabinene **18.55%**
beta-pinene **15.55%**
gamma-terpinene **5.1%**
safrole **2%**
alpha-terpineol **1%**
eugenol **0.2%**
isoeugenol **0.2%**

Caution: People taking antidepressant medication should avoid frequent use of Nutmeg oil until further evidence shows that there is no drug/oil interaction.

Large dosages of nutmeg can be psychotropic and toxic.

Why it works

Alpha-pinene is a mild antiseptic and also a warming agent, making Nutmeg oil useful in liniments and for stiff muscles.

Terpinen-4-ol is an antibacterial agent, though at less than 10% in the oil, it may not have significant effects.

Myristicin's odor contributes to the oil's uplifting, spicy Nutmeg scent.

Myrtus communis

Myrtle

Myrtle is a medium-sized shrub originating in North Africa but cultivated in the Mediterranean. It belongs to the Myrtaceae family; other members include Eucalyptus *(Eucalyptus globulus)* and Tea Tree *(Melaleuca alternifolia)*. It produces fragrant flowers and leaves, and the fruits are sometimes used as a spice in cooking. In Italy and Greece, a traditional cough syrup is made from its leaves, and it is used in some commercial cough preparations.

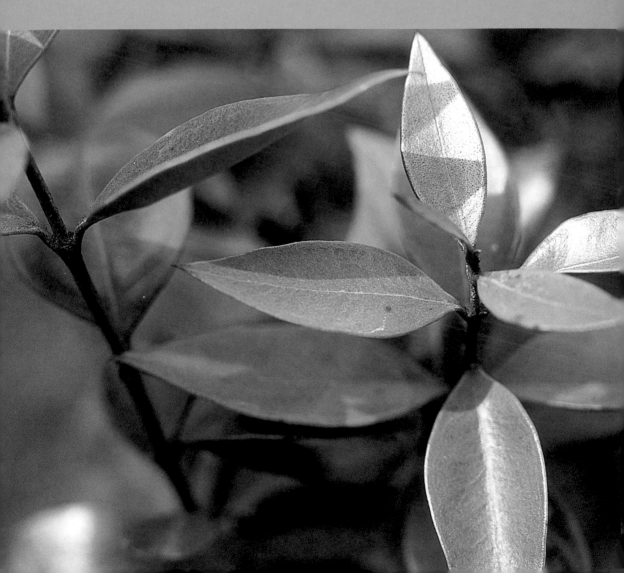

Myrtle oil is extracted from the leaves and twigs by steam distillation, and is usually a pale yellow to greenish color, with a fresh scent reminiscent of Eucalyptus. There is a wide variation in oil quality, the most prized being that from the Mediterranean island of Corsica. There seems to be confusion over the naming of the oils, with some companies labeling it Red Myrtle and others Green Myrtle. It is advisable to smell a sample before buying, to make sure that you are getting the one you like.

Traditional aromatherapy uses

Myrtle oil is mainly used in European aromatherapy, and is excellent as a milder version of Eucalyptus oil (*E. globulus*, see page 88). It is commonly used for bronchial complaints in children and elderly people, having both decongestant and antibacterial properties. It is also used for muscular aches and pains.

Ailments and remedies

Painful coughs and bronchitis Add 2 drops of Myrtle oil to a ceramic bowl of hot tap water and inhale the vapors, covering the head with a towel. Inhale through nose and mouth alternately to coat the respiratory surfaces. Repeat 3–4 times a day, and preferably return to bed after each inhalation to prevent becoming chilled.

Muscular aches and pains Add 5 drops of Myrtle oil to 1 tablespoon of vegetable oil and massage gently into the affected area. Cover the part with a warm compress or towel to help relieve any stiffness.

Why it works

Myrtenyl acetate is likely to be responsible for Myrtle oil's relaxing reputation and gives the oil its herbaceous sweet scent.

1,8-cineole and **alpha-pinene** contribute to the oil's usefulness in treating respiratory conditions, particularly congestion of the lungs and sinuses. Both compounds are also warming when applied to the skin, so it is good for muscular aches and pains.

Alpha-terpineol contributes mild antibacterial properties along with alpha-pinene, which would also help alleviate respiratory infections.

Caution: If Myrtle oil smells very strongly like Eucalyptus oil, it means it contains a high percentage of 1,8-cineole. If this is so, do not take Myrtle oil internally, and avoid its use in inhalations for people with asthma or for children under 12 months old (see *Eucalyptus globulus* cautions).

Myrtle oil should be used when fresh. It can be kept up to 6 months at room temperature and a maximum of 12 months in the refrigerator.

Myrtle
Spain
(wild)

Active constituents

myrtenyl acetate **35.9%**
1,8-cineole **29.9%**
alpha-pinene **8.1%**
alpha-terpineol **4.1%**

Other known constituents

limonene **7.5%**
methyl eugenol **2.3%**
carvacrol **0.6%**
myrtenol **0.58%**
linalyl acetate **0.53%**
isobutyl isobutyrate **0.4%**

Ocimum basilicum

Basil {Sweet Basil}

This aromatic plant from the family Lamiaceae, to which many of the Mediterranean herbs belong, is a main ingredient in leaf form in many Italian pasta sauces, including the Genoese Pesto. Another species, *Ocimum sanctum*, is sold as Holy Basil or sometimes under its ayurvedic name, *Tulsi*. Tulsi is used in Thai cuisine, and is not to be confused with *Ocimum basilicum*.

The essential oil of Basil is steam distilled from the leaves and flowering parts, and is produced in many regions of the world. The best known is Reunion oil, produced in the Comoros, a tiny group of islands near Madagascar in the Indian Ocean. Reunion oil is preferred by flavorists and perfumers due to its strong aniseed odor. European Basil oil smells more floral and herbaceous than Comoros Island Basil.

Traditional aromatherapy uses

Basil oil is used to help relieve menstrual pain or the pain of intestinal cramping. Basil is often vaporized as a study aid, usually in a blend with Rosemary and Lemon oils.

Ailments and remedies

Basil	Active constituents	Other known constituents
Comoros Islands (Methyl chavicol)	methyl chavicol **85%** linalool **0.96%**	1,8-cineole **3.25%** para-cymene **2.7%** methyl eugenol **1.3%** eugenol **0.45%** p-methoxycinnamaldehyde **0.4%**, spathulenol **0.12%**
France (Linalool)	linalool **38.2%** methyl chavicol **16.4%** beta-caryophyllene **7%**	eugenol **5.1%** methyl (E)-cinnamate **4.7%** alpha-terpinyl acetate **4.5%** 1, 8-cineole **3.5%** terpinen-4-ol **2.5%** gamma-cadinene **2.28%**

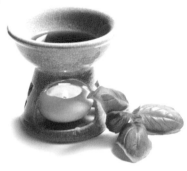

Menstrual cramps Add 5 drops of Basil oil (methyl chavicol) to a basin containing about 3 pints (2 liters) of hot water. Soak a small hand towel in it and apply to abdomen or lower back as a warm compress. Repeat as often as necessary to provide relief, but without adding more oil.

Intestinal discomfort (flatulence, stress-induced constipation)
Add no more than 5 drops of Basil oil (methyl chavicol) (in case of skin sensitivity) to a tablespoon of vegetable oil (olive oil will do if you have nothing else). Massage into the abdomen in a clockwise direction starting at the bottom left. This follows the route of the large intestine and will provide relief from the pressure.

Mental stress Add 3 drops of Basil oil (linalool) to a vaporizer in an average-sized bedroom, or up to 6 drops for a large living area. The smell will invigorate initially, and then calm the nervous system and promote restful sleep. Do not vaporize Basil (linalool) oil when you will be driving!

Why it works

Methyl chavicol, (also known as estragole) has a strong aniseed odor and flavor. It also has antispasmodic properties and probably accounts for Sweet Basil oil's use in treating menstrual cramps and constipation. The strong odor of methyl chavicol makes Sweet Basil oil useful in stimulating alertness.

Linalool has a calming and sedative effect. Sweet Basil oils from different locations have different ratios of linalool and methyl chavicol components, which affects their therapeutic properties. Reunion Basil oil, from the Comoros Islands, would be more suitable as an antispasmodic, whereas European Basil, with a higher content of linalool, would be more suitable for mental stress. Oils from the same botanical species that have marked chemical differences are known as "chemotypes."

Beta-caryophyllene found in the European Basil has anti-inflammatory properties.

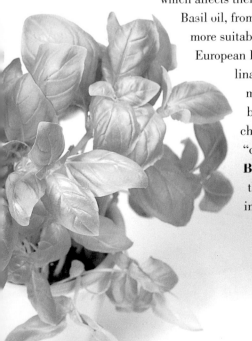

Origanum majorana Sweet Marjoram

Sweet Marjoram oil comes from the Lamiaceae family of plants, along with the majority of essential-oil-producing herbs, such as Rosemary, Sage, Lavender, Basil, Thyme, and Oregano. The alternative botanical name is *Marjorana hortensis*. There are several species of Marjoram, which are often cultivated for garden purposes.

Sweet Marjoram should not be confused with *Origanum vulgare*, which produces a reddish essential oil similar to *Thymus vulgaris*.

The oil is steam distilled from the leaves and flowering tops of the plant, and is a clear to pale yellow, with an odor similar to Tea Tree oil, but sweeter. Aromatherapists consider that the oil can be helpful in lowering blood pressure.

Traditional aromatherapy uses

Sweet Marjoram essential oil is mainly thought of as a relaxing oil. It can also be applied as an antibacterial agent, although some sources suggest it is more useful for its antispasmodic properties.

Ailments and remedies

High blood pressure Add 3 drops of Sweet Marjoram oil to a vaporizer and vaporize for a couple of hours. If you dislike the smell, blend the oil with 2 drops of a citrus oil. Stop using the oil if you feel drowsy.

At the end of the day, add 3 drops of Sweet Marjoram oil to a warm bath, and relax in it for 15 minutes, preferably with low light levels. Do not discontinue any medication you may be taking, but monitor any effects in consultation with your doctor.

Cuts and abrasions Add 5 drops of Sweet Marjoram oil to a bowl of warm water, and use to bathe the cut or abrasion. Repeat twice a day.

Why it works

Terpinen-4-ol has been shown to have broad-spectrum antibacterial properties. Terpinen-4-ol is also the major active component in Tea Tree oil (*Melaleuca alternifolia*, see page 108). It is also a mild local anesthetic.

Para-cymene may antibacterial, but can be irritating on the skin.

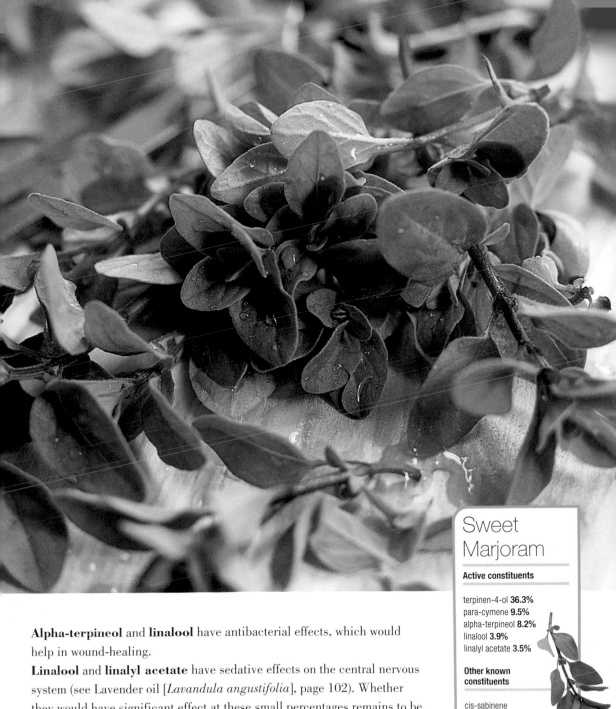

Alpha-terpineol and **linalool** have antibacterial effects, which would help in wound-healing.

Linalool and **linalyl acetate** have sedative effects on the central nervous system (see Lavender oil [*Lavandula angustifolia*], page 102). Whether they would have significant effect at these small percentages remains to be shown.

None of the known constituents has been shown to have specific blood pressure lowering activity, which is one of the more common uses of Sweet Marjoram oil in aromatherapy. However, further research may well reveal an active ingredient.

Caution: Para-cymene may cause irritation in people with sensitive skins, though the percentage of this constituent varies from different sources. If in doubt, test a small patch of skin with 3 drops of Marjoram oil in 1 teaspoon of vegetable oil before using it on a larger area.

Sweet Marjoram

Active constituents

terpinen-4-ol **36.3%**
para-cymene **9.5%**
alpha-terpineol **8.2%**
linalool **3.9%**
linalyl acetate **3.5%**

Other known constituents

cis-sabinene hydrate **15.9%**
bicyclogermacrene **2.5%**
beta-caryophyllene **2%**

Pelargonium graveolens
Geranium

The name geranium, derived from the *Geranium* genus, has been applied to the closely related *Pelargonium* genus for so long that it is now common usage. An essential oil known as Zdravetz oil is commercially produced from the Bulgarian *Geranium macrorrhizum*, but its odor is entirely unlike the lovely rose-like scent of the oil from the *Pelargonium* species. *Pelargonium* plants are indigenous to countries in southern Africa, although there are some species in India and Australia.

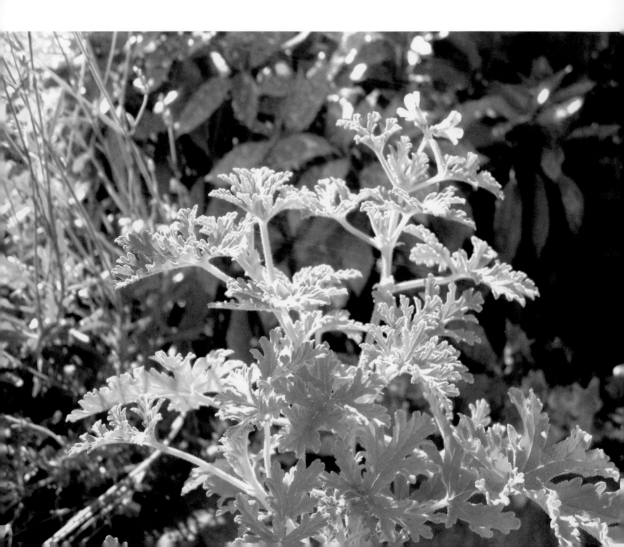

There is some confusion over the different species, which is not surprising since the plants readily hybridize, and some essential oil suppliers use less common botanical names. *Pelargonium graveolens*, *P. capitatum*, and *P. roseum* all produce a rose-scented essential oil. A commercial name for the Geranium oil from Réunion island in the Indian Ocean is the hybrid *P.* x *asperum*. It is usually referred to as Geranium Bourbon oil from the time when the island was a colony of France. It is the most highly prized of the rose-scented *Pelargonium* oils. The oil of *P. odoratissimum* has either an apple-like or a minty odor.

The pale greenish-yellow essential oil is primarily extracted by steam distillation from the leaves and stems of the plants. The flowers do not have an essential oil, despite the flowery scent of the plant. One of the main uses of Geranium oil is in perfumery and cosmetics.

Traditional aromatherapy uses

Geranium oil is used as an antibacterial in wound healing and the treatment of acne and pimples. It is also indicated as a soothing aid for conditions such as shingles and other diseases that cause neuralgia (nerve pain). It is also thought of as a "balancer" for conditions where hormones have got out of balance, particularly in women.

Ailments and remedies

Oily skin and acne Put 1 or 2 drops of Geranium oil onto clean fingers and dab directly onto oily areas of the face and pimples. Alternatively, put 5 drops of Geranium oil into a bowl of warm water, squeeze a clean facecloth into it, then apply with gentle pressure all over the face. This can also be a nice pick-me-up at the end of a heavy day's work.
Shingles Put 3–5 drops of essential oil into a cool or warm bath (whichever you tolerate best) and let your body rest in the water while you inhale the lovely fragrance of the oil. Think calm thoughts and let the tension slide off into the water.

Why it works

Citronellol, **geraniol**, and **linalool** are antibacterial and have mild anesthetic properties on the skin.
Citronellol and **geraniol** combine to give the rose-like odor, and are the main components of Rose oil (*Rosa damascena*, see page 138). Geranium oil is sometimes used to adulterate or extend Rose oil due to this similarity.
Citronellyl formate and **geranyl formate** contribute to the sweetness of the odor and may contribute calming properties.
Isomenthone and **menthone** add a minty note to the odor and may also contribute antispasmodic effects for intestinal muscles. They could also give Geranium possible cooling effects on the skin.

Geranium Bourbon

Active constituents

citronellol **21.2%**
geraniol **17.45%**
linalool **12.9%**
citronellyl formate **8.37%**
geranyl formate **7.55%**
isomenthone **7.2%**
menthone **1.5%**

Other known constituents

guaia-6,9-diene **3.9%**
geranyl butyrate **1.3%**
citronellyl butyrate **1.26%**
cis-rose oxide **0.64%**
furopelargone A **0.37%**
2-phenylethyl tiglate **0.43%**
trans-rose oxide **0.21%**

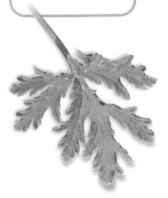

Pimpinella anisum
Aniseed

Aniseed is a member of the Umbelliferae family, like Sweet Fennel *(Foeniculum vulgare)*. The seeds are used in cooking by several cultures, in both sweet and savory dishes. Candied aniseed and fennel seeds are served after a hot curry meal to aid the digestion and sweeten the breath.

The alcoholic Greek drink ouzo is flavored with the main constituent of aniseed oil, anethole, which gives the essential oil its characteristic taste. Aniseed oil is also used in confectionery and certain soft drinks.

The oil is available from many different countries, including India and Spain, and is produced by steam distillation of the seeds. The striking looking star-shaped Star Anise seed pods, illustrated here, are used in Asian savory dishes, The essential oil produced from Star Anise is very similar to aniseed.

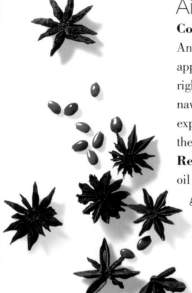

Traditional aromatherapy uses
Aniseed oil is used to relieve spasms associated with indigestion, flatulence, and menstrual cramping. It can be used alone or with Fennel oil.

Ailments and remedies
Constipation and flatulence Add 10 drops of Aniseed oil, or 5 drops of Aniseed and 5 drops of Sweet Fennel oil to 1 tablespoon of vegetable oil and apply in sweeping clockwise strokes to the belly. Start at the bottom of the right-hand side of the belly and sweep up to the ribs, then across above the navel, and down to the bottom left. Repeat the motion as often as necessary, experimenting with varying pressure, as required. If the constipation is severe, the entire belly may need extremely gentle handling.

Respiratory congestion Put 1 drop of Aniseed oil, 1 drop of Peppermint oil (*Mentha piperita*, see page 116) and 1 drop of Eucalyptus oil (*Eucalyptus globulus*, see page 88) into a bowl of hot water, and inhale the vapors through the nose and the mouth alternately. A towel covering the head will keep the vapors in.

Why it works
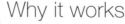
Anethole is the major component and significant odor in Aniseed oil. In tests, anethole is known as an

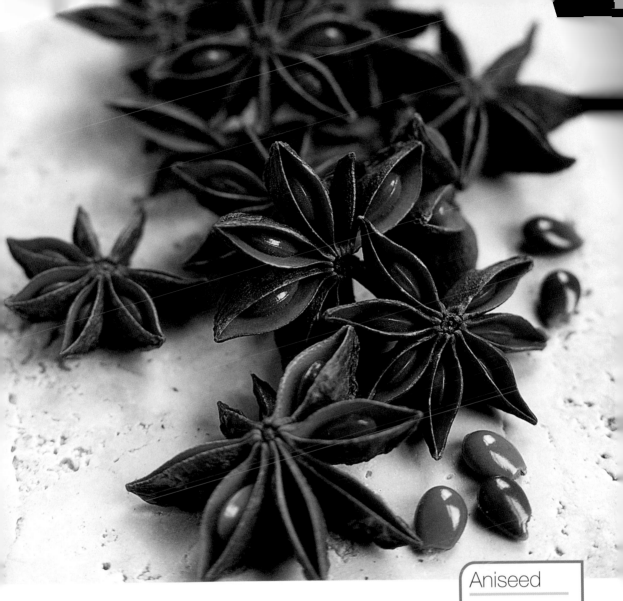

antispasmodic for muscle tissue, in particular the intestines and uterus. Bronchial constriction may also be reduced by inhalation of oils containing anethole. Some experts suggest that anethole may have mild estrogenic properties.

Anisaldehyde and **anisalcohol** contribute to the odor of the oil, but it is not known whether or not they have any beneficial effects.

Caution: Anethole may act as a mild estrogen and in high doses may affect estrogen-dependent cancers. However, the amounts absorbed during an abdominal massage or inhalation as described above are extremely unlikely to pose any risks. If concerned, avoid use of Aniseed oil with endometriosis and breast or ovarian cancers.

Do not use Aniseed oil on people with liver disease, or babies under 12 months old, and avoid use on women who are pregnant or breastfeeding.

Aniseed

Active constituents

Anethole **96%**
anisaldehyde **0.6%**
anisalcohol **0.4%**,

Active constituents

Limonene **1.6%**
(Z)-anethole **0.36%**
methyl chavicol **0.3%**
linalool **0.26%**
coumarins **1%**

Pinus pinaster

Pine

There are many different species of Pine tree, most of which produce aromatic resins and have fragrant needles. Both the resins and the needles can be distilled to produce terpenoid oils, but only the needle oil is used in aromatherapy.

Turpentine oil has been used as an antibacterial agent, and as a remedy for sprains and muscular aches. Other residues from the distillation of the resin are pitch and tar. Pine tar has been used as a remedy for eczema and other skin diseases.

Oil from the Scotch Pine (*P. sylvestris*) has similar qualities to *P. Pinaster* but should not be used directly on the skin.

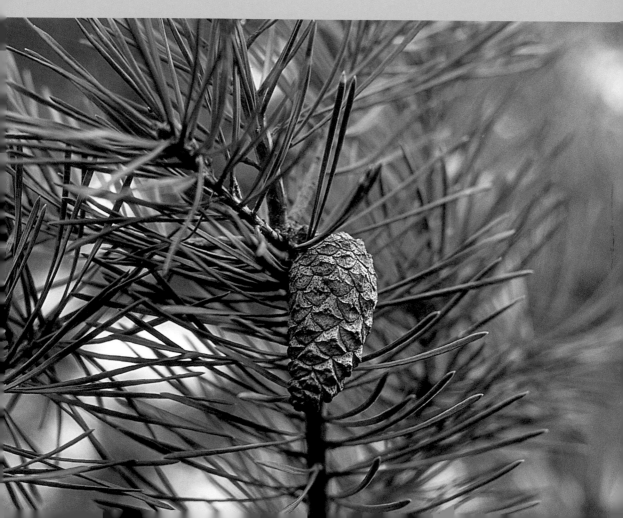

Traditional aromatherapy uses

Pine oil (*P. pinaster*) and Scotch pine oil (*P. sylvestris*) are traditionally used as an expectorant for respiratory infections. *P. pinaster* oil is used to relieve muscular aches and pains. It is also thought to be a diuretic and a stimulant for the circulation.

Ailments and remedies

Bronchitis and chest coughs Add 3 drops of Pine (*P. pinaster*) oil to a ceramic bowl of hot tap water and inhale through the nose and mouth, covering the head with a towel. If the inhalation causes too much coughing, stop and wait for a minute or two, then resume.

Muscular aches and pains Add 5 drops of Pine (*P. pinaster*) oil to 1 tablespoon of vegetable oil, and massage into the affected area.

Why it works

Alpha- and **beta-pinene** give *P. pinaster* and *P. sylvestris* mild antibacterial properties, and also make them useful for the relief of muscular aches and pains. They also contribute the typical pine odor.

Beta-caryophyllene although in small amounts, may contribute anti-inflammatory properties, helping relieve tight chest coughs and sore muscles.

Delta-3-carene on its own has been shown to cause skin allergies in humans. At less than 5%, it is unlikely to pose much of a problem in Pine oil, but Scotch Pine oil (*P. sylvestris*) may cause problems for people with sensitive skins.

Limonene adds a fresh lemon note to the odor, which probably contributes to its use in disinfectants.

Alpha-terpineol is present in only small amounts, but would nevertheless contribute antibacterial properties.

> **Caution:** Do not use Scotch Pine oil on the skin, as it can contain significant amounts of delta-3-carene (about 20%). This compound has been shown to initiate skin allergies in some people. People with allergic asthma should possibly avoid use of Scotch Pine oil in inhalations as well.

Pine	Active constituents	Other known constituents
Pinus pinaster	alpha-pinene **44.1%** beta-pinene **29.5%** beta-caryophyllene **3.5%** delta-3-carene **3.4%** alpha-terpineol **1.3%**	myrcene **4.6%** limonene **3.2%** germacrene D **2.1%** cadinene **0.9%**
Pinus sylvestris (Scotch Pine)	alpha-pinene **42%** delta-3-carene **20.5%** limonene **5.2%**	cadinene **4.76%** germacra-1-(10)-E,5E-dien-4-ol **1.89%** T-cadinol **0.56%** bornyl acetate **0.12%**

Piper nigrum
Black Pepper

Black Pepper oil is extracted from the dried unripe fruits of *Piper nigrum*, a vine that grows in India and other parts of Asia. The dried fruits, or peppercorns, have been used as a savory spice for over 4,000 years by both Eastern and Western cultures.
If the fruits ripen before drying, they yield white pepper, but no essential oil is commercially available from white peppercorns.

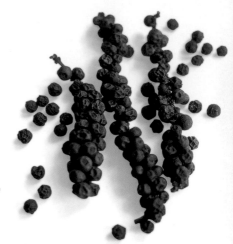

Most of the essential oils derived from spices are reputed to have an effect on digestion. This is probably because the cultures in which the spices are traditionally used in cooking practice a holistic healing system, in which food is viewed as medicine. Ayurvedic (traditional Hindu) medicine, in particular, recommends the addition of different spices to food depending upon the presenting conditions. Some sources suggest Black Pepper can be used if the liver is sluggish or the stomach is not producing enough acid.
P. nigrum is not to be confused with the other plants known as peppers or bell peppers, from the *Capsicum* genus or the Californian Pepper Tree (*Schinus molle*).

Black Pepper oil is extracted either by steam distillation or by CO_2 extraction. The steam-distilled oil has a lemony or pine-like smell. The CO_2 extract smells more like freshly crushed black pepper.

Black Pepper

Active constituents (steam distilled)

beta-caryophyllene **34.6%**
delta-3-carene **16%**
limonene **14.5%**
alpha- and beta-pinene **10%**

Active constituents (steam distilled)

alpha-copaene **3%**
delta-elemene **2%**
alpha-cubebene **0.2%**,
torreyol **0.2%**

Traditional aromatherapy uses

Black Pepper oil is used as a rubefacient (warming) agent. A rubefacient is useful in many situations, such as muscular aches and pains. People suffering from conditions such as chronic fatigue often have cold hands and feet and may benefit from a brisk rub with a vegetable oil blend containing Black Pepper oil.

Ailments and remedies

Cold hands and feet Add 5 drops of Black Pepper oil (steam distilled) to 2 tablespoons of vegetable oil and massage the legs, starting at the feet and moving up to the thighs. If you do the massage at bedtime, put socks on to keep the oils on the skin; if you do it in the morning, cover the feet for the first few hours of the day. The hands can be massaged as shown on page 32.
Feverish aches and pains If a cold or influenza causes you to shiver and ache, massage the aching parts with the same blend as above to help yourself feel warmer and less shivery.

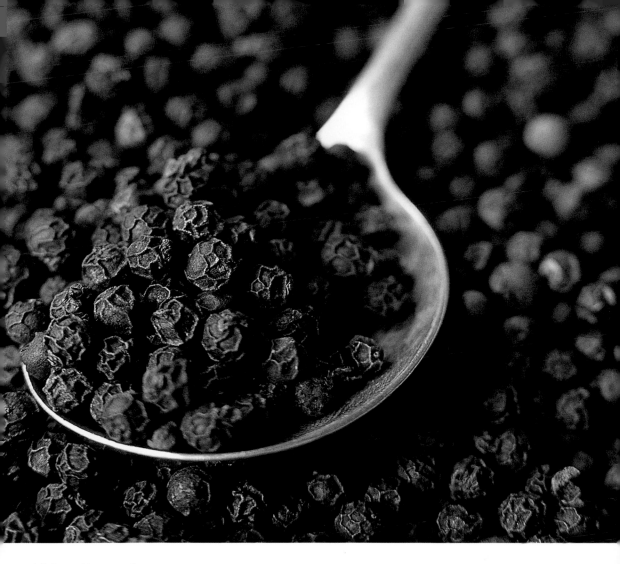

Why it works

Beta-caryophyllene is usually about a third of Black Pepper oil's make up. It has anti-inflammatory properties and gives the oil its warm, spicy aroma. **Delta-3-carene** on its own is known to cause skin allergies, but in the presence of the other components of the oil, and in the small quantities used in aromatherapy, it seems not to have this effect. However, the percentage of delta-3-carene can vary. If it is more than about 15–20%, do not use the oil on the skin.

Limonene and **alpha-** and **beta-pinene** contribute fresh lemon and pine notes to the oil's odor. Limonene has been shown to stimulate bile flow, and the pinenes are used as mild antiseptics and liniments.

The CO_2 extract is preferred by flavor technologists because it captures a greater percentage of the pungent flavor compounds which are not extracted in steam distillation. These compounds are also likely to be more irritating on the skin and mucous membranes, so the CO_2 extract is not used on the skin.

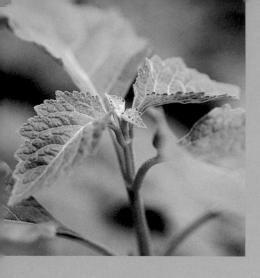

Pogostemon cablin

Patchouli

Patchouli is a tropical rainforest shrub, which produces fragrant blossoms, leaves, and twigs. Surprisingly, it comes from the same botanical family (Lamiaceae) as many of the herbaceous oils. Patchouli oil was used extensively in the 1960s as a "hippie" perfume, and has a rich, woody fragrance with incense-like overtones, which masks other odors.

Patchouli oil has been used in Asian cultures as an aphrodisiac, and as a moth repellent in woolen garments and carpets exported from India. It is used in the perfumery industry as a base for Oriental fragrances, and acts as a fixative for other more volatile aroma compounds.

Patchouli oil is produced in Indonesia and in other parts of Asia. It is steam distilled from the dried leaves, and is usually available as a fairly viscous, deep orange-red oil. The oil becomes a more intense orange as it ages, and the older oil is preferred in the perfume industry for its more complex, mellow odor. You can purchase a clear, pale yellowish-green oil, which smells similar, but most people favor the orange-red oil.

Traditional aromatherapy uses

Patchouli oil is used for inflammatory skin conditions, such as eczema, psoriasis, dandruff, and tinea. It is an astringent, so it is also helpful in cases where an inflammation is wet or oozing. Patchouli is useful in helping to reduce anxiety, and in what some aromatherapists term the "grounding" of people who are vague or distracted.

Ailments and remedies

Itchy skin Add 3 drops of Patchouli oil to 1 teaspoon of vegetable oil, or use undiluted. Apply to the affected area up to three times a day, and monitor the itching and inflammation. Three drops of Lavender oil (*Lavandula angustifolia*, see page 102) can be added to the blend, if preferred.

Mental distraction Vaporize 3 drops of Patchouli oil in a vaporizer, or wear 1 drop of Patchouli oil as a perfume on the collarbones to help focus and "ground" mental energies.

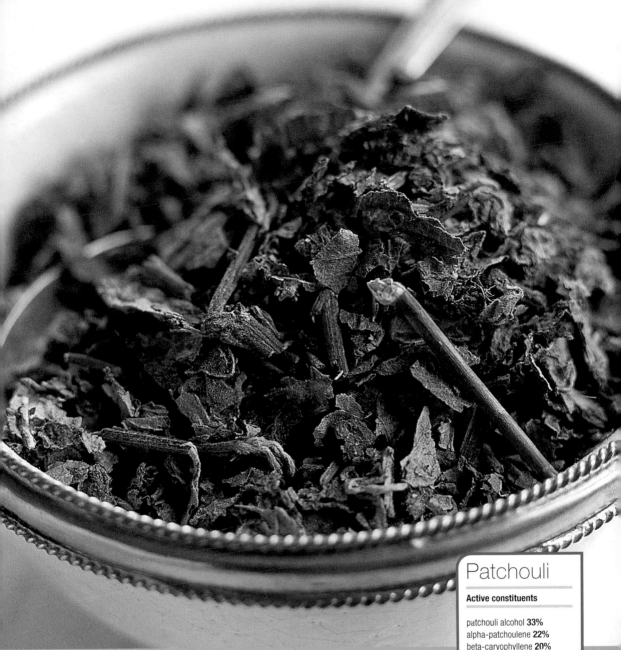

Why it works

Patchouli alcohol, and **alpha-** and **beta-patchoulene**, may contribute to the anti-itching properties of the oil.

Beta-caryophyllene has known anti-inflammatory effects.

Beta-elemene has been shown to have antitumoral activity, and with the other anti-inflammatory constituents may account for Patchouli's traditional use in skin care.

Patchouli

Active constituents

patchouli alcohol **33%**
alpha-patchoulene **22%**
beta-caryophyllene **20%**
beta-patchoulene **13%**
beta-elemene **6%**

Other known constituents

norpatchoulenol **1%**
pogostol **0.4%**
caryophyllene oxide **0.3%**
delta-guaiene **0.3%**,
patchoulenone **0.05%**
patchouli oxide **0.05%**
patchouli pyridine **0.05%**

Rosa damascena

Rose

Roses have been valued as fragrant and beautiful flowers for many centuries and in many cultures, and have been extensively cultivated and hybridized. The hybrids usually lose their scent in exchange for exotic colors. The red fruit of the plant, the rose hip, is used as a source of Vitamin C and rose hip syrup can provide a gentle boost for the immune system.

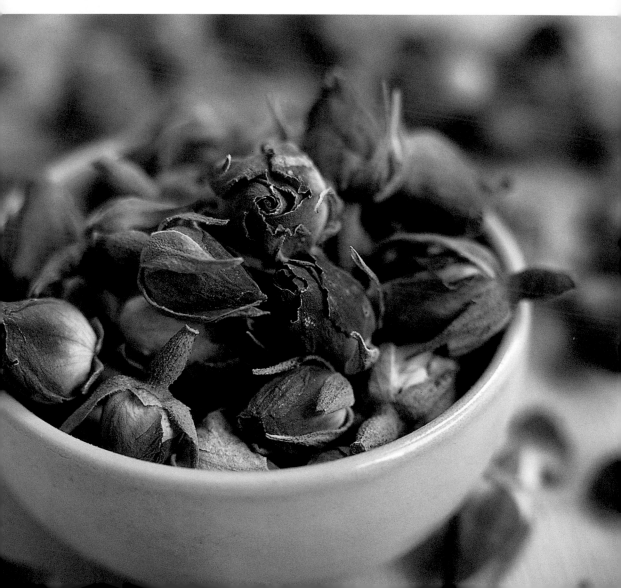

The species of rose typically used in aromatherapy is *Rosa damascena*, although the oil from *R. centifolia* is also produced commercially. As with many floral oils, the flowers produce only tiny quantities of oil per blossom, so Rose oil is traditionally very expensive. The flowers also need special treatment: handpicking, followed by extraction with solvents to obtain the concrete (or absolute), which is a waxy solid at room temperature; and finally, an extraction of the concrete to obtain the oil—also known as an otto. The color of the otto varies, but is usually a somewhat viscous yellow.

Bulgaria and Turkey produce the best-quality Rose oil, with its characteristic, almost geranium-like scent, which differs from the smell of the flower because of the concentration of the odor. Egypt and Morocco produce an oil that smells more like the rose itself, but which has a different chemical composition.

Traditional aromatherapy uses

Rose oil is traditionally considered useful for gynecological and women's hormonal problems, and the mood states that tend to accompany them. It is also used in skincare preparations for its ability to soften and restore youthful qualities to the skin, helping to reduce the redness of capillaries.

Ailments and remedies

Dry and red skin Add 3 drops of Rose oil to 1 teaspoon of Jojoba oil, or use a prediluted oil. Massage into the face, neck, and hands, and enjoy the beautiful fragrance.

Grief or loss Wear 1 drop of Rose oil as a daily perfume to help you through periods of grief and loss.

Why it works

Citronellol, geraniol, and **nerol** contribute to Bulgarian Rose oil's geranium-like scent. Bulgarian Rose oil has a long tradition of use in beauty care, which is confirmed by the activities of these compounds. They have antibacterial properties and also may help constrict the tiny blood capillaries that redden the cheeks.

2-phenyl ethyl alcohol has not been researched for its therapeutic effects, but it may be found to have an effect on mood. It has the sweet typical rose odor that you smell when first smelling a red or pink rose.

Farnesol has anti-inflammatory and antibacterial properties.

Stearopten waxes found in Bulgarian Rose otto have not been investigated for therapeutic properties, but they may contribute to the usefulness of Rose otto for dry skin.

Rose

Bulgaria
Otto

Active constituents

citronellol **33.4%**
geraniol **18%**
nerol **5.9%**
2-phenyl ethyl alcohol **1.3%**

Other known constituents

stearopten waxes **24%**
linalool **2.1%**
eugenol **1.5%**
farnesol **0.87%**
methyl eugenol **0.5%**
geranial **0.5%**
cis-rose oxide **0.4%**
3-hexenal **0.26%**
carvone **0.22%**
trans-rose oxide **0.4%**
beta-damascenone **0.05%**

Egypt
Otto

Active constituents

2-phenyl ethyl alcohol **37.9%**
geraniol **15.8%**
citronellol **12.6%**
nerol **4%**
farnesol **6.3%**

Other known constituents

linalool **2.2%**
eugenol **1.2%**
alpha-ionone **1%**

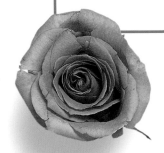

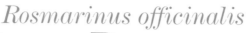

Rosmarinus officinalis
Rosemary

Rosemary comes from the Lamiaceae family, whose members include the majority of essential oil-producing herbs, such as Sage, Lavender, Basil, Thyme, and Oregano.

Rosemary has been used for centuries in religious and magical ceremonies, sometimes in place of incense. Rosemary oil is steam distilled from the leaves and flowering tops of the plant, and is a clear, colorless to pale yellow. Powdered Rosemary wood was thought to be a preventive against tooth decay. A vinegar made from the leaves was used as a cure for coughs. An infusion of the leaves, applied as a hair rinse, was reputed to control dandruff and to prevent baldness by stimulating the hair follicles.

Rosemary
Spain
Camphor CT

Active constituents

alpha-pinene **22%**
camphor **17%**
1,8-cineole **17%**

Other known constituents

verbenone **4%**
borneol **2%**
bornyl acetate **1.5%**
terpinen-4-ol **1.5%**
alpha-terpineol **1.5%**

Tunisia
Cineole CT

Active constituents

1,8-cineole **51.3%**
camphor **10.6%**
alpha-pinene **10%**

Other known constituents

borneol **7.7%**
alpha-terpineol **3.9%**
terpinen-4-ol **1%**
bornyl acetate **0.8%**
alpha-humulene **0.7%**
verbenone **0.05%**

Traditional aromatherapy uses

Rosemary is used for its stimulant effects upon memory and concentration. It is also useful as an expectorant in respiratory diseases, and to alleviate muscular aches and poor circulation.

Ailments and remedies

Poor concentration Add 2 drops of Rosemary (camphor type) oil to a vaporizer and vaporize for 1 hour in the workplace or study environment. It is recommended to alternate use of different oils with Rosemary if you are working intensively for an entire day.

Poor circulation and muscular aches Add 3 drops of Rosemary oil (cineole type) to 1 tablespoon of vegetable oil and rub vigorously into the soles of the feet to stimulate the circulation. Apply the blend to any particular aching spot and massage to aid penetration of the oil.

Why it works

The three types of Rosemary oil available are known as chemotypes (CT) because they differ in their chemical composition. The North African cineole CT contains high proportions of 1,8-cineole and alpha-pinene. The camphor CT, of Spain and France, contains higher proportions of camphor and borneol than the cineole chemotype. The verbenone CT has similar constituents, but higher levels of verbenone and bornyl acetate.

1,8-cineole and **alpha-pinene** give Rosemary oil the odor of of Eucalyptus oil (*Eucalyptus globulus*, see page 88), and in high proportions similar

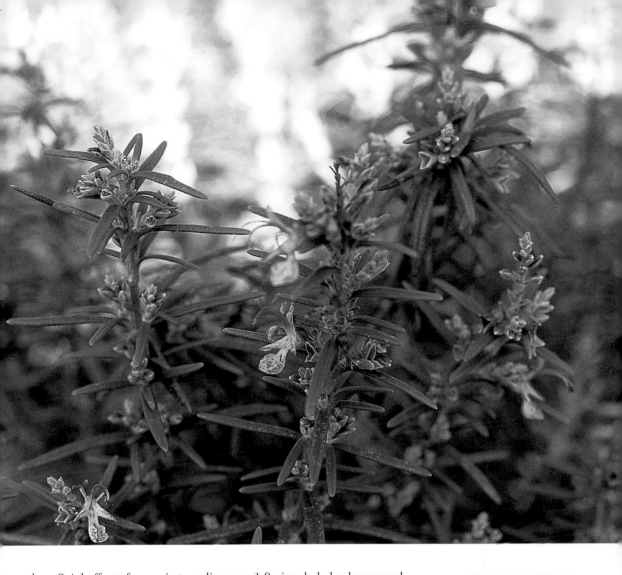

beneficial effects for respiratory diseases. 1,8-cineole helps loosen and remove excess mucus, and alpha-pinene adds antibacterial properties.

Camphor gives Rosemary oil its camphoraceous earthy smell. Camphor has warming effects on the skin, and makes Rosemary oil useful in liniments and to treat muscular aches and pains. Pure camphor cubes available from drug stores as moth repellents are sometimes eaten by children. It can cause neurotoxic effects ranging from confusion and nausea to convulsions, depending on the amount eaten. The quantity of camphor in Rosemary oil is unlikely to have any neurotoxic effects with the amounts recommended for use in aromatherapy. In fact, camphor in aromatherapy doses may contribute to the cognition-stimulating effects of Rosemary.

Verbenone and **bornyl acetate** characterize the other chemotype (CT) of Rosemary oil. The therapeutic properties of these compounds have not been determined, but the oil is considered less powerful in effect than the other two chemotypes. The other two chemotypes are more commonly used in aromatherapy.

Caution: Do not take any type of Rosemary oil internally in case it has high camphor content, which may cause neurotoxic effects. Rosemary oil should be avoided during pregnancy, because of its neurotoxicity. Some sources say that Rosemary oil should not be inhaled or used on the skin by people with epilepsy as the camphor content may trigger a seizure.

Salvia sclarea

Clary Sage

Clary Sage oil is derived from the leaves of the furry-leaved *Salvia sclarea* plant. There are several fragrant *Salvia* species, which produce different oils and should not be confused. Clary Sage is the most commonly used *Salvia* oil in aromatherapy. The aroma of Clary Sage is very distinctive, with a sweet,spicy, muscat-like odor.

Clary Sage

**Active constituents
(steam distilled)**

linalyl acetate **49%**
alpha-terpineol **3%**
geraniol **2.4%**
linalool **24%**
sclareol **0.31%**

**Other known constituents
(steam distilled)**

germacrene D **3%**
geranyl acetate **2.5%**
3-hexenol **0.2%**
spathulenol **0.03%**

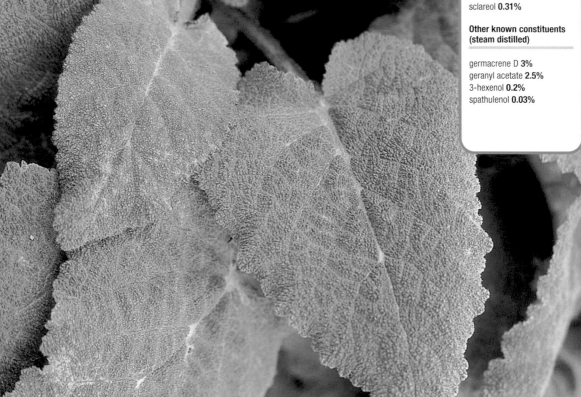

The seeds of Clary Sage form a frothy mucilaginous mass when soaked in water, and according to some sources, this was used for extracting small particles from the eye—hence clary, from "clear eye." This mucilaginous mass was also applied to tumors and swellings, and for the drawing out of thorns and splinters. In early 19th-century England, the herb was used to add bitterness when brewing beer. Clary Sage beers were renowned for producing a euphoric intoxication, followed by a severe headache.

Clary Sage oil is extracted by two methods: steam distillation and solvent extraction. The steam-distilled oil is used in aromatherapy, whereas the solvent extract is used as a flavoring in tobacco and some muscatel wines (presumably adding to the intoxicating effect) and as a fixative in perfumery.

Traditional aromatherapy uses

Clary Sage oil is traditionally used as an antispasmodic for menstrual pain, and as a regulator of women's hormones. Some sources recommend it for use during childbirth, since it is supposed to accelerate labor, though this has not been proved experimentally. It has also been used as an antidepressant and a relaxant, particularly for panic and nervous hysteria.

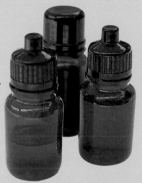

Ailments and remedies

Menopausal hot flashes Use the same treatment as for menstrual pain, or wear the oil as a perfume, dabbing 1–2 drops behind the ears and on the nape of the neck.

Menstrual pain and premenstrual stress Add 5 drops of Clary Sage oil to 1 teaspoon of vegetable oil and massage the lower back and abdomen in gentle circular movements.

Nervous exhaustion Run a deep warm bath at bedtime, and add 3 drops of Clary Sage oil to the bath just before you get in. Alternatively, anoint the midline of your body with 3 drops of oil before getting into the bath. Lower the lights, or use only a candle, turn on the answering machine, and relax, using your favorite meditation or mantra.

Why it works

Linalyl acetate and **linalool** are the same major components found in Lavender oil (*Lavandula angustifolia*, see page 102) and Bergamot oil (*Citrus bergamia*, see page 64). They have sedative and relaxing effects, which make all three oils useful for the treatment of nervous anxiety and stress. These may also be the constituents responsible for the antispasmodic effects of Clary Sage oil. **Linalool**, **alpha-terpineol**, and **geraniol** have antibacterial properties.

Sclareol contributes a musky ambergris-like aroma. It has a structure similar to some steroid hormones. It may be the constituent responsible for the reputed effects of Clary Sage on women's menstrual problems and premenstrual tension.

> **Caution:**
> Most aromatherapists recommend avoiding use of Clary Sage oil if you will be drinking alcohol. Some people have experienced a severe hangover doing so, when usually they wouldn't get a hangover.

Santalum album

Sandalwood

Sandalwood has been used for centuries as a wood for carving sacred objects, for incense, and for its thick gorgeous oil, which is used as a natural perfume base for many Indian perfumes. Traditionally it was grown in the state of Mysore (now Karnataka) in southern India, but demand outstripped supply, and the state's plantations can no longer meet the world's requirement for pure sandalwood oil.

The oil only develops its prized odors when the tree is at least 30 years old, and sustainable management practices were not implemented in time. Another species of Sandalwood, *Santalum spicatum*, native to Australia, produces an oil that is similar to the Mysore Sandalwood oil, although it has a fresher, somewhat lemony top note. Both types of Sandalwood oil are used as a remedy for sore throats, though the Australian Aboriginals use an infusion of the inner bark, not the oil. Sandalwood oil of both types also has a reputation for treating sexually transmitted diseases, though orthodox treatments should not be discontinued while using it.

The thick, yellowish oil is steam distilled from the heartwood of the tree, and has a characteristic warm, balsamic, woody scent. As in the case of Patchouli, the odor mellows and becomes more complex as the oil matures.

Sandalwood
India

Active constituents

cis-alpha-santalol **50%**
cis-beta-santalol **20.9%**
epi-beta-santalol **4.1%**

Other known constituents

alpha-santalal **2.9%**
cis-lanceol **1,7%**
trans-beta-santalol **1.5%**
spirosantalol **1.2%**
santalenes **1.7%**
cis-nuciferol **1.1%**
beta-santalal **0.56%**
eka-santalals **0.08%**

Traditional aromatherapy uses

Sandalwood is used as a form of spiritual protection by therapists who practice on that level. It is also traditionally associated with male energy and is used as an aphrodisiac for men. Its anti-inflammatory action makes it useful for dry and inflamed skin and for sore and dry throats. It is also used for pruritis and other forms of genito-urinary infections.

Ailments and remedies

Itchy skin Sandalwood oil can be applied undiluted to areas of itchy skin, but since it is expensive, you may prefer to dilute it in vegetable oil (5 drops to 1 teaspoon of vegetable oil), or to add 3 drops to a warm bath. Adding 3 drops of Sandalwood oil to an unscented base cream can make a lovely soothing cream for everyday use.

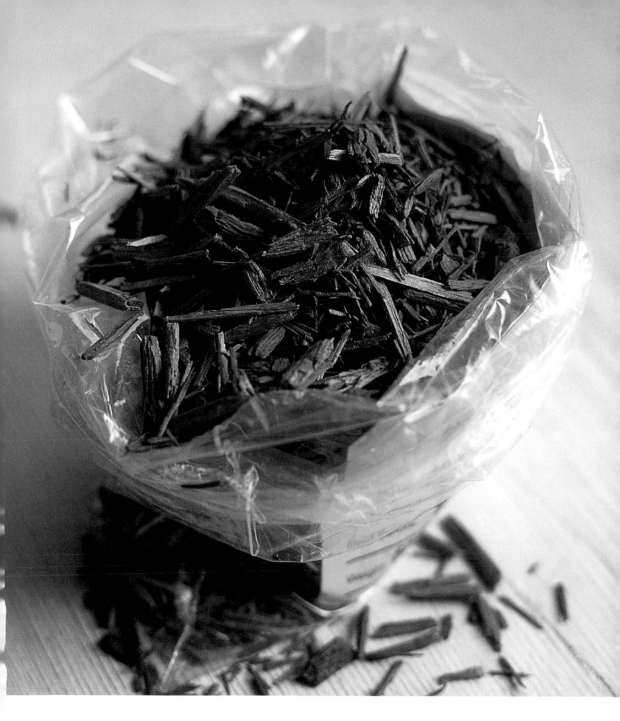

Genito-urinary infections and itching Add 3 drops of Sandalwood oil to
a shallow warm bath and soak the affected area in it for about 10 minutes.
Using a finger or cotton-tipped applicator, dab undiluted Sandalwood oil
onto the affected areas, especially if they are raw or inflamed.

Why it works

The **santalol compounds** are the major component of the oil, and are
thought to contribute to its anti-inflammatory properties.

Styrax benzoin
Benzoin

Trees from the Styraceae family are found in the rainforests of Sumatra, Java, Laos, and Vietnam. Skilled forester-farmers make shallow cuts in the trunks of the trees to harvest the resin without killing the trees. Siam Benzoin (*Styrax tonkinensis*) is considered to be the most valuable of the Styrax resins and is only found in certain forest regions of northern Laos. Sumatra Benzoin (*S. benzoin* or *S. paralleloneurus*) is more commonly available.

Benzoin resin has been used in herbal cough medicines in Asia and Europe for hundreds of years. Words formerly used for resin were balsam and balm, which also mean "agents that soothe." The resin can be burned as an incense when placed on a charcoal block, and the smoke from Benzoin has a very pleasant sweet and warm odor. It blends well with Frankincense and Myrrh resins, and is often sold in a mixture for meditation.

The odor of the Siam Benzoin is described as balsamic or vanilla-like, whereas the Sumatra Benzoin, while still balsamic, has a harsher, more bitter aroma. Unlike the resins of Frankincense and Myrrh, no true essential oil is produced from the resin. To liquify it, an ethanolic tincture or absolute of the resin is often made, or it is liquified with a range of other solvents, including some vegetable oils. Benzoin is used as a fixative in perfumery and as a preservative in cosmetics, because the coniferyl esters have high boiling points and are antifungal and antibacterial.

Traditional aromatherapy uses

Benzoin tincture is used in steam inhalations for persistent respiratory infections, especially catarrh and bronchitis. It is also used for skin infections, such as scabies and ringworm, and conditions such as dandruff, psoriasis, or tinea. The affected area is swabbed with Benzoin tincture.

Ailments and remedies

Catarrh and bronchitis Add 5 drops of Benzoin tincture to a large bowl of steaming water and inhale the vapors. Cover the head with a towel to gain the full effect.

Itchy skin Add 5 drops of benzoin tincture or resinoid to 1 tablespoon of vegetable oil and rub gently into the affected area. You can add 2 drops of German chamomile (*Matricaria recutita*) to the blend if you like.

Caution:
Some people are sensitive to Benzoin. If skin irritation occurs, wipe off and then rinse vigorously with cold running water.

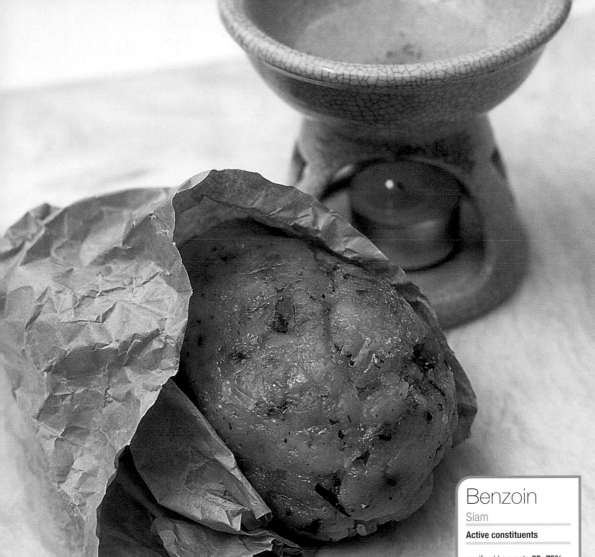

Why it works

Coniferyl benzoate and **coniferyl cinnamate** are responsible for the breaking down of mucous in conditions like catarrh and persistent bronchitis. Enzymes in the lung and sinus linings convert the molecules into compounds, which have mild irritant and antibacterial properties. These compounds also evaporate slowly on the skin, and make Benzoin useful as a fixative in perfumery.

Benzoic acid is often used as a preservative in cosmetics. It can cause skin irritation or allergies in some people.

Benzyl benzoate kills *Ascarides* mites, which cause scabies and dust allergies. Benzoic acid and the other benzyl compounds may well contribute to this action.

Vanillin gives Siam Benzoin oil its delicious vanilla odor, which the Sumatra Benzoin usually lacks.

Benzoin

Siam

Active constituents

coniferyl benzoate **65–75%**
benzoic acid **10–12%**
benzyl benzoate **(varying %)**
vanillin **0–2%**

Other known constituents

benzyl cinnamate and other benzyl compounds **(varying %)**

Sumatra

Active constituents

coniferyl cinnamate **55–70%**
cinnamyl alcohol **5–9%**

Other known constituents

benzo-resinol, phenyl propyl alcohol **(varying %)**

Thymus vulgaris

Thyme (Sweet thyme)

Thyme comes from the Lamiaceae family of plants, like many essential oil-producing herbs, such as Sage, Lavender, Basil, Rosemary, and Oregano. Thyme leaf tea is used to alleviate colic, and also as a gargle for sore throats. Thyme oil is extracted from the leaves of the plant by steam distillation.

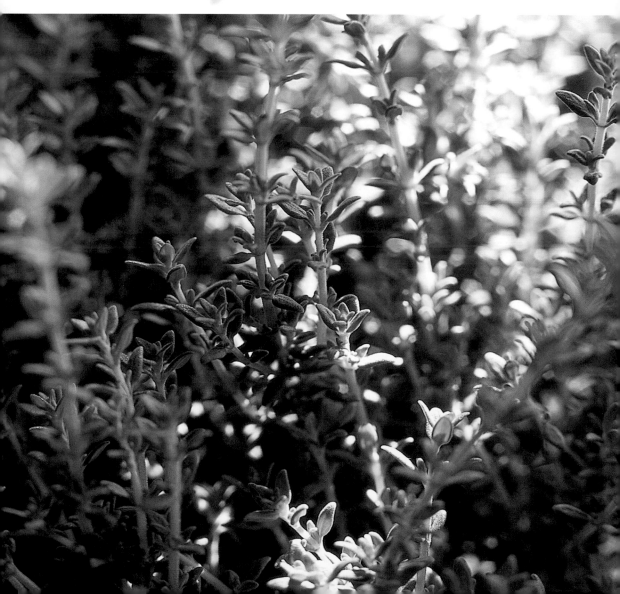

Though there are many different species and chemotypes (CT) of Thyme, most aromatherapists prefer to use the linalool chemotype of *Thymus vulgaris*, because it is mild on the skin. Thyme CT linalool should be a clear pale yellow color.

Traditional aromatherapy uses

The pale yellow linalool chemotype (sometimes known as Sweet Thyme) is used as an effective antibacterial oil, and as a warming oil in a massage blend.

Ailments and remedies

Arthritic pain Add 3 drops of Thyme oil (linalool) to 1 tablespoon of vegetable oil, and massage the painful area.

Boils and infected pimples Use a cotton-tipped applicator to dab Thyme linalool onto a boil or infected pimple to help fight the infection.

Cold hands and feet Use the same blend as for arthritic pain and rub vigorously into the soles of the feet and the lower legs, using strokes that move upward toward the heart. Squeeze the calves and the feet, as if to squeeze the blood upward. Massage the hands as shown on page 32.

Why it works

Thyme oils can range from pale yellow to red-brown in color. The red-colored oils contain substantial amounts of carvacrol, which, although a strong antibacterial agent, is a skin and mucous membrane irritant. Most aromatherapists consider red Thyme oils hazardous for use in aromatherapy. The pale yellow Thyme oils have high percentages of milder compounds like linalool, geraniol, geranyl acetate, borneol, or cineole. The linalool chemotype of *Thymus vulgaris* is preferred due to its pleasant lavender-like odor and safety on the skin.

Linalool and **linalyl acetate** are both noted as sedative compounds. However, Thyme Linalool is not noted for its sedative effects, possibly because it is mainly used as an antibacterial agent.

Linalool, terpinen-4-ol, and **thymol** work together to provide a strong, but safe antibacterial effect, and make Thyme Linalool useful for skin and respiratory infections. It is one of the best oils to use for fighting bacteria, and can be used with Tea Tree oil (*Melaleuca alternifolia*, see page 108).

Caution: If Thyme Linalool causes skin irritation, wipe off immediately and rinse vigorously with cold running water.

Do not use Thyme oil that is red or brown in color because it may cause skin irritation.

Thyme
Italy (linalool chemotype)

Active constituents

linalool **77%**
linalyl acetate **8%**
terpinen-4-ol **4%**
thymol **2.2%**

Other known constituents

beta-caryophyllene **2.8%**
para-cymene **2%**
carvacrol **trace**

Vanilla planifolia, V. fragrans
Vanilla

Vanilla is a sweet flavoring that is rated more popular than chocolate. It comes from an orchid indigenous to Mexico, and is cultivated in many parts of the world. The pale yellow flower must be hand fertilized when grown outside the Mexican rainforests, and yields a long green bean-like pod. The pods are harvested and cured according to a time-honored practice until they assume a dark, leathery consistency with the characteristic vanilla odor.

An alcoholic extract of the cured pods is sold as vanilla extract, which is used around the world in ice creams, confectionery, sweet bakery, and perfumery. Vanilla was considered by the Aztecs to be an aphrodisiac, and it was also used to counteract venomous bites and prevent headaches. Another species, *V. tahitiensis*, is grown in Tahiti, and produces a floral-scented extract. The *V. planifolia* extract used in aromatherapy is derived by evaporating the alcohol off the alcoholic extract. Vanilla extract is also produced by carbon dioxide extraction, and other forms of solvent extraction.

Traditional aromatherapy uses

Some sources suggest the use of vanilla as a remedy for anger, tension, and irritability; others confirm the traditional use of vanilla as an aphrodisiac. Its use in "comfort" foods suggests that it may be useful in stimulating appetite.

Ailments and remedies

Irritability Use 1 drop of Vanilla extract as a personal perfume, either on a tissue tucked into a bra strap, or on the inside of your collar. Alternatively, add 3 drops of vanilla to a vaporizer, blending with a citrus oil, such as Mandarin, if preferred, to curb the intense sweetness of the vanilla.

Lack of sexual desire Add 1 drop of Vanilla extract to a warm bath and inhale the warm sweet aroma, allowing your sensual nature to come out and play. Vanilla blends well with 1 drop of Ylang ylang and 1 drop of Sandalwood—also noted as aphrodisiac oils. Subtlety is important in the art of love, so don't overdo the number of drops!

Sweet food cravings Take a sniff from the Vanilla bottle every time you crave sweet food. It could help to curb your appetite.

Why it works

Vanillin gives the extract its characteristic odor. From its chemical structure, vanillin could be expected to be a good antibacterial compound. Apart from its delicious taste, perhaps this is one of the reasons it is used to flavor sweet foods. One research study examined the potential of vanillin to prevent seizures, and found that vanillin showed mild anti-convulsive effects. The extract is often adulterated with synthetic vanillin which is produced from fermentation of wood chips, but the synthetic on its own does not have the full richness of the odor provided by the 130 or so trace constituents in the extract.

4-hydroxybenzaldehyde may enhance the binding of the brain transmitter, gamma-amino butyric acid (GABA), thus creating a general calming effect. However, the research is in very early stages and the effects remain to be demonstrated conclusively.

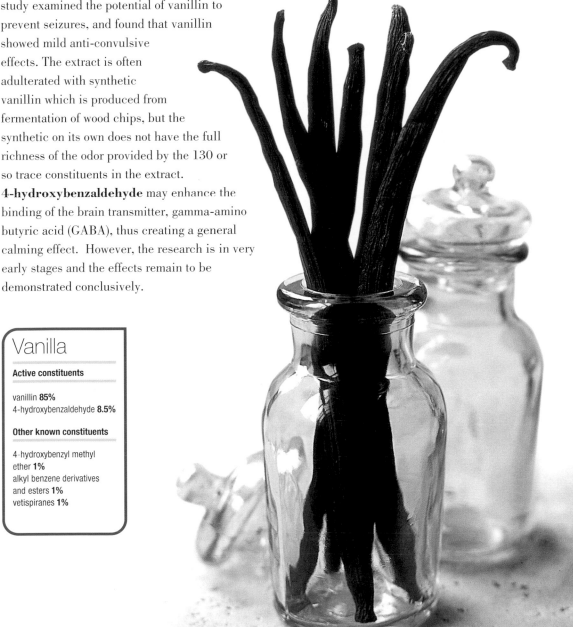

Vanilla

Active constituents

vanillin **85%**
4-hydroxybenzaldehyde **8.5%**

Other known constituents

4-hydroxybenzyl methyl
ether **1%**
alkyl benzene derivatives
and esters **1%**
vetispiranes **1%**

Vetivera zizanoides

Vetiver

Vetiver is a tropical grass grown in several Southeast Asian countries, which has fragrant leaves and roots. The therapeutic uses vary from country to country, but a paste or decoction of the roots is widely reputed to be a remedy for headaches, arthritis, and rheumatism. Decoctions of the roots are also used to soothe fevers. They are also used for their insect-repellent properties, and recent research is proving that some components of Vetiver oil are helpful in repelling termites.

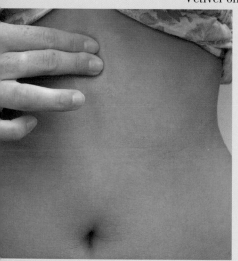

Massaging the solar plexus with Vetiver oil can help relieve nervous anxiety.

Vetiver oil is extracted from the chopped roots by steam distillation, and yields a dark brown, viscous oil with an earthy, woody, smoky scent, similar to that of Patchouli. Vetiver oil is used in perfumery as a fixative, and as a base for certain "woody" perfumes. The oil is also known as "khus" oil.

Traditional aromatherapy uses

Vetiver oil is primarily used for its calming and so-called "grounding" effect on emotions. Similarly to Patchouli oil (*Pogostemon cablin*, see page 136), it is used to relieve itchy skin, and should also produce a soothing effect on aching joints.

Ailments and remedies

Confusion and nervous anxiety With a finger, put 1 drop of undiluted Vetiver oil onto the solar plexus area, just below the bottom of the sternum, and gently massage the oil in. Rub the remaining oil from your finger onto your palms and inhale deeply from them. Blending 1 drop of Lavender oil with the Vetiver oil will sweeten the aroma.
Muscular tension and joint pain Add 3 drops of Vetiver oil to 1 tablespoon of vegetable oil and gently massage the tense or painful area. If there is time, ask someone to do a full body massage to help reduce the tension.
Itchy skin Add 5 drops of Vetiver oil to 1 teaspoon of vegetable oil, and apply gently to the affected area. Repeat morning and evening or as needed.

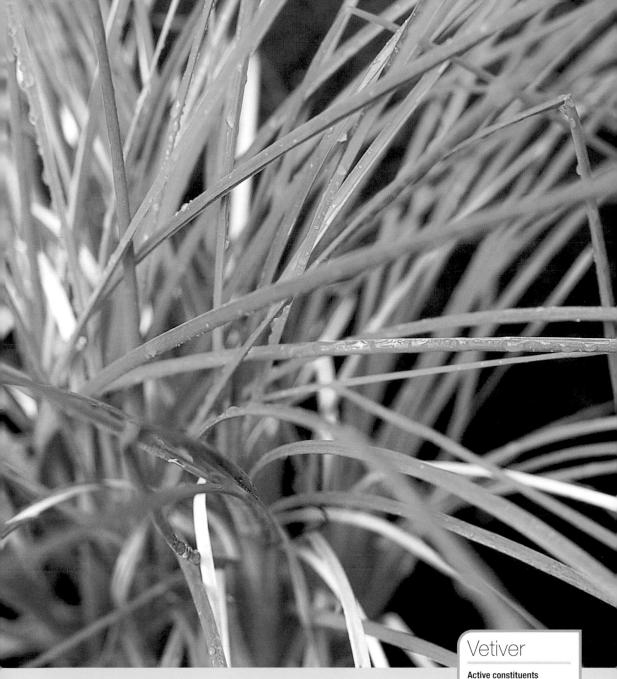

Why it works

All the compounds in Vetiver oil are large molecules that give the oil a
low volatility and make it useful as a perfumery fixative.
Vetiverol, **vetivene**, and **alpha-vetivol** share a similar structure to
compounds in other oils that have known anti-inflammatory activity. It is
likely that they contribute to the traditional antiarthritic properties of
Vetiver oil, and also help reduce the itchiness of itchy skin.
There is not much scientific evidence for the therapeutic effects of the
individual compounds in Vetiver oil at this stage.

Vetiver

Active constituents

vetiverol **50%**
vetivenes **20%**
alpha-vetivol **10%**

Other known constituents

vetivones **10%**
khusimol **1%**
khusimone **1%**
vetiselinene **1%**
vetispirenes **2%**
vetiazulene **0.1%**

Zingiber officinale

Ginger

Ginger oil is extracted from the fleshy roots (rhizomes) of the *Zingiber officinale* plant. Along with Galangal and Cardamom, Ginger is a spice from the Zingiberaceae family. Ginger is common all over China, India, and other parts of Asia, and has been used for centuries in many different cultures as a medicine and as a therapeutic food.

The Japanese serve pickled ginger with their raw fish dishes to prevent possible food poisoning; the Indians and Chinese regard Ginger as a warming and fortifying aid to the circulation; and the English picked up on its digestive qualities by eating candied ginger after dinner to aid digestion. Recent trials demonstrate its usefulness in relieving nausea, and as a relief for the pain of arthritis and other inflammatory conditions. The oil is extracted either by steam distillation, which produces a pale yellow oil, or by CO_2 extraction, which yields a deep orange-yellow oil. The CO_2 extract is notably more pungent than the steam-distilled oil.

Traditional aromatherapy uses

Ginger oil is traditionally used in aromatherapy to alleviate nausea in pregnancy and travel sickness, and to alleviate the spasms of colic. It is also used to stimulate circulation and "warm up" a sluggish metabolism.

Ailments and remedies

Nausea Add 5 drops of Ginger oil to 1 teaspoon of vegetable oil and massage over the stomach area just under the rib cage.
Alternatively, make a thermos bottle of ginger tea by pouring boiling water onto about 1 in. (2.5 cm) of finely chopped fresh gingerroot and allowing it to steep for about 5 minutes. Drink a cup when you feel nauseous.

Sluggish feeling Add 5 drops of Ginger oil to 1 tablespoon of vegetable oil and massage vigorously into the arms and legs, using brisk brushing strokes toward the heart.

Caution:
If Ginger oil or CO_2 extract of Ginger cause skin irritation, wipe off immediately and rinse vigorously with cold running water. To avoid risk of skin irritation, always dilute Ginger oil in vegetable oil before applying it to the skin.

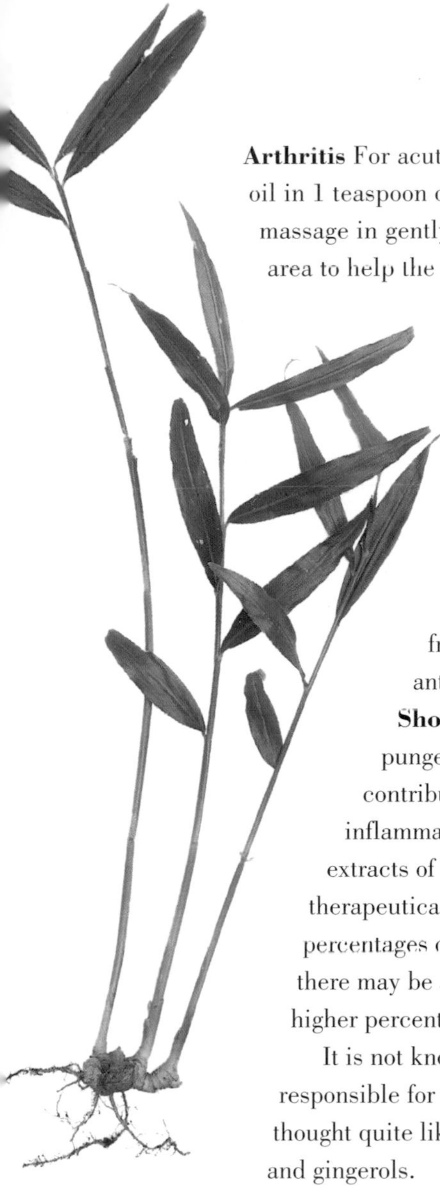

Arthritis For acute pain, apply up to 5 drops of Ginger oil in 1 teaspoon of vegetable oil directly to the joint and massage in gently. If possible, apply a heat pack to the area to help the oil to penetrate the joint.

Why it works

Curcumene and **alpha-zingiberene** have anti-inflammatory effects that would contribute to the use of Ginger oil for arthritis.

Citral and **geraniol** give the oil its fresh lemon-like odor and add to antibacterial effects of the oil.

Shogaol and **gingerol** give the oil its pungent ginger aroma, and probably contribute most to the warming and anti-inflammatory properties of the oil. CO_2 extracts of Ginger are likely to be more powerful therapeutically, as they contain higher percentages of shogaols and gingerols. However, there may be added risk of skin irritation with higher percentages of shogaols and gingerols.

It is not known exactly which compounds are responsible for the antinausea effects of ginger, thought quite likely it is the shogaols and gingerols.

Ginger
China (steam distilled)

Active constituents

curcumene **16.3%**
alpha-zingiberene **14.2%**
citral **4%**
geraniol **1.7%**
shogaol **(trace)**
gingerol **(trace)**

Other known constituents

beta-sesquiphellandrene **10.6%**
bisabolenes **10.51%**
zingiberenol **1.4%**
citronellol **1.2%**
beta-eudesmol **0.9%**
2-undecanone **0.3%**
6-methyl-5-hepten-2-one **0.2%**
hexanal **0.05%**
decanal **0.04%**

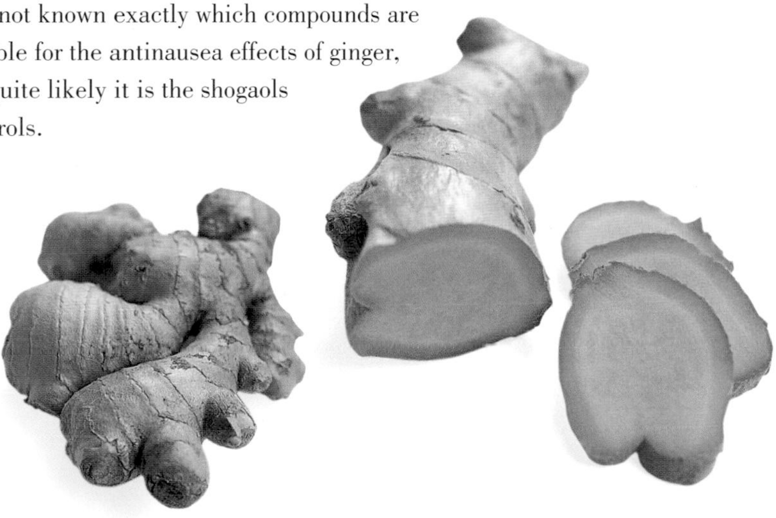

Glossary

Aldehyde: Essential-oil constituent with antifungal and possibly irritant properties. Mostly found in lemon-scented and citrus oils.

Antispasmodic: Relieving contraction of muscles— skeletal, intestinal, and bronchial.

Astringent: Drying, or causing contraction of tissues. Useful against overproduction of secretions.

Chemotype: Botanically identical plants with different ratios of essential-oil constituents. For example, Basil (methyl chavicol chemotype) has about 80% methyl chavicol. By contrast, Basil (linalool chemotype) has

about 40% linalool and only 40% methyl chavicol.

Cold-pressing: See Expression

Compress: A cloth soaked in water containing essential oils, to provide heat or cold to an area of the body in addition to the essential oils.

Constituent: A chemical component of an essential oil.

CT: Chemotype.

Esters: Essential-oil constituents, some of which have antispasmodic and relaxing properties, e.g. linalyl acetate in *Lavandula angustifolia* oil.

Ethers: Essential-oil constituents with intestinal antispasmodic and euphoric properties.

Expression: Method of extracting essential oils from citrus peel by crushing the peel to squeeze the oils out. Preferred to steam distillation method.

Furocoumarin: Component of Bergamot oil that causes photosensitization.

Gas chromatography: Technique for analyzing essential oils, separating out the different constituents using their varying chemical characteristics.

Genus: Major plant classification group and the first of a plant's botanical names, e.g. *Lavandula* in *Lavandula angustifolia.* Often abbreviated to the initial letter when comparing two species of the same genus, e.g. *L. angustifolia.*

Hydrosol/hydrolat: Water collected after steam distillation of essential oils. Can be fragrant and is often used in cosmetics, or even in cooking, e.g. rose water.

Infused oil: Vegetable oil in which plant material is soaked for up to two weeks, so that the plant constituents are dissolved in the oil. A form of solvent extraction.

Ketone: Essential-oil constituents with

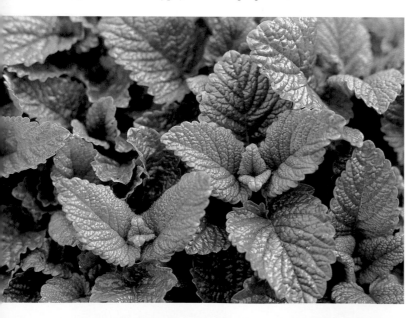

antispasmodic and mucous-drying properties.

Lipid: Fat-soluble substance.

Lipophilic: Dissolving in fats, oils, and organic solvents.

Monoterpenes: Essential-oil constituents with mild stimulating properties.

Monoterpenols: Essential-oil constituents with antibacterial and mild analgesic properties.

Oxide: Only one oxide constituent is commonly found in essential oils: 1,8-cineole. It has expectorant and mucolytic (mucous-releasing) effects.

Phenols: Essential-oil constituents with strong antibacterial and antifungal properties.

Photosensitization: A reaction of furocoumarins to UV in sunlight that may cause inflammation of the skin.

Phytotherapy: Treatment of disease with plant extracts; herbal medicine.

Receptor: A large protein molecule embedded in the membrane of a cell, which enables the cell to receive chemical information. The analogy of a "lock and key" is often used to describe this mechanism. The receptor is the lock, and the chemical that binds to it is the key.

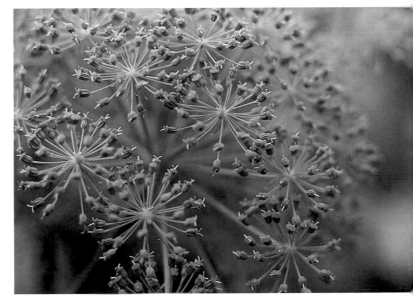

Rubefacient: Causing redness and warmth on the skin; increasing bloodflow to an area.

Sesquiterpenes and *sesquiterpenols:* Essential-oil constituents, often with a woody aroma and anti-inflammatory properties.

Solvent extraction: Method of extraction of essential oils that uses solvents, such as hexane or ethanol, to extract the oils, in contrast to steam distillation. Plants with low essential-oil yield are often solvent-extracted, Rose and Jasmine, for example.

Species: The last botanic name of a plant, e.g. *angustifolia* in *Lavandula angustifolia.*

Several species can belong to the same genus.

Steam distillation: Method of extracting essential oils from plant material using steam. The most widely used means of extraction.

Tincture: Alcoholic extract of herbal plant material.

Var.: Abbreviation of the Latin *varietas* meaning variety. Used in the botanic name, e.g. *Cananga odorata* var. *genuina.*

Vasoconstrictive: constricting the blood vessels.

Virucidal: Disables or kills viruses.

Index

Abies alba (White Fir) 42-43
A. balsamea (Balsamic Fir) 42
aches and pains 89, 104, 134
Achillea millefolium (Yarrow) 38, 44-45
acne 36, 63, 66-67, 129
Amomum elettaria see Cardamom oil
Angelica archangelica (Angelica) 46-47
Angelica Root oil 46-47
Aniba rosaeodora (Rosewood) 48-49
Aniseed oil 79, 90, 130-131
ankles, swollen 70, 80-81
Anthemis nobilis (Roman Chamomile) 39, 50-51, 92, 106
anxiety 51, 61, 65, 152
appetite, lack of 74, 100
aromachology 22
aromas, effects of 22-23
arthritis 37, 100, 110-111, 149, 154-155
asthma 52, 56
athlete's foot 38, 83
ayurvedic medicine 13, 58, 76, 134

Basil oil 22, 23, 114, 124-125, 126, 140, 148
in massage 28
Bay Laurel oil 100-101
Bay oil 100
Benzoin tincture 16, 38, 146-147
Siam 146, 147
Bergamot oil 39, 49, 63, 64-65, 66, 68, 72, 143
in massage 33
Bigarade oil *see* Petitgrain oil
"blue" moods 55, 66, 70, 72, 74
body odor 85
boils 149
Bois-de-Rose *see* Rosewood oil
Boswellia carterii (Frankincense) 52-53, 56, 76
B. frereana 52
B. serrata 52
bowel spasms 91
bronchitis 98, 104, 113, 123, 133, 146
bruises 92
burns 36, 102

Cade oil 96
Cajuput oil 38, 59, 100-111, 112, 113
Cananga odorata var. *genuina* (Ylang ylang) 39, 54-55
Canarium luzonicum (Elemi) 56-57, 76
C. muelleri (Queensland Elemi) 56
C. schweinfurthii 56
Caraway oil 119
Cardamom oil 58-59
Cardamomum elettaria (Cardamom) 58-59
Carum carvi (Caraway) 119
catarrh 146
Cedarwood oil, Virginia 85, 98-99
in massage 33
cellulite 36, 70, 74, 80-81
Chamaemelum nobile see Anthemis nobilis
Chamomile *see* German Chamomile oil; Moroccan Chamomile; Roman Chamomile oil
Cinnamomum camphora (Chinese Ho plant) 48
circulation, poor 36, 140
Citratus flexuosus see Lemongrass oil
Citronella oil 83, 84, 86-87, 115
Citrus aurantifolia (Key Lime) 66
C. aurantium var. *amara* (Neroli) 39, 60-61, 73
(Petitgrain) 39, 62-63
C. bergamia (Bergamot) 39, 63, 64-65, 143
C. latifolia (Lime) 66-67
C. limonum (Lemon) 39, 68-69
C. paradisii (Grapefruit) 70-71, 36
C. reticulata (*C. deliciosa*) (Mandarin) 39, 72-73
C. sinensis (Sweet Orange) 73, 74-75
Clary Sage oil 44, 142-143
Clove oil 100
cold hands and feet 134, 149
cold sores 115
colds 38, 58, 104, 110, 113
colic 79, 119
Commiphora myrrha (Myrrh) 36, 56, 76-77

concentration, poor 39, 140
confusion 152
constipation 125, 130
Coriander oil 78-79
Coriandrum sativum (Coriander) 78-79
coughs 38, 58, 89, 110, 123, 133
cramps 45
Cupressus sempervirens (Cypress) 36, 80-81
Curry Plant *see* Immortelle oil
cuts and abrasions 36, 45, 56, 76, 126
Cymbopogan citratus (Lemongrass) 82-83, 84, 86, 109, 115
C. martini (Palmarosa) 83, 84-85, 86
C. nardus (Sri Lankan Citronella) 86
C. winterianus (Citronella) 83, 84, 86-87, 115
Cypress oil 36, 52, 80-81

depressive moods 39, 55, 65, 66, 72, 74, 94, 120
dry skin 36, 49, 52, 85, 139

Elemi oil 56-57, 76
emotional instability/ vulnerability 39, 49
energy, lack of 72-73, 83
essential oils
additions to 20
analysis 20, 21
extraction 14-15
nature 12-13
physiological effects 18-19
properties 18
quality 21
Eucalyptus globulus (Eucalyptus) 58, 59, 88-89, 100, 101, 111, 112, 113, 122, 130, 140-141
E. radiata 88
Eucalyptus oil 58, 59, 88-89, 100, 101, 111, 112, 113, 122, 123, 130, 140-141
Eugenia caryophyllus (Clove) 100
eyes, sore 107

Fennel oil, Sweet 44, 58, 79, 90-91, 130

Fir oil
Balsamic 42
Douglas 42
White 42-43
flatulence 58, 91, 125, 130
focus, lack of 69, 136
Foeniculum vulgare var. *dulce* (Sweet Fennel) 58, 79, 90-91, 130
fragrance oils 16, 20
Frankincense oil 52-53, 56, 57, 76, 146
in massage 26, 27

genito-urinary infections 145
Geranium macrorrhizum (Zdravetz oil) 128
Geranium oil 36, 85, 128-129
Bourbon 129
German Chamomile oil 23, 36, 37, 50, 51, 79, 99, 106-107, 146
in massage 28, 32
Ginger oil 58, 93, 154-155
Grapefruit oil 36, 66, 68, 70-71, 72
grief and loss 139

headache 116
hedonic response 22
Helichrysum italicum (*H. angustifolium*) (Immortelle) 92-93
hemorrhoids 80
herbal teas 16-17
high blood pressure 126
hot flashes 143

Immortelle oil 92-93
indigestion 79, 116, 119
influenza 38, 89, 104, 110
insect bites and stings 36, 102, 106
insect repellent 86
insomnia 65, 102
intestinal spasms 61, 116
irritability 72, 150
itchy skin 36, 98, 106, 136, 144, 146, 152

Jasmine oil 23, 61, 73, 94-95
in massage 27
Jasminum grandiflorum (Jasmine) 61, 73, 94-95
J. paniculatum 94
J. sambac 94, 95

jet lag 72-73
joints, swollen 96
Juniper oil 36, 96-97, 120
Juniperus communus (Juniper)
    36, 96-97, 120
J. mexicana 98
J. oxycedrus (Cade) 96
J. sabina (Savin) 96
J. virginiana (Virginia
    Cedarwood) 98-99

Laurus nobilis (Bay Laurel)
    100-101
*Lavandula angustifolia (L.
    officinale)* (Lavender)
    19, 36, 37, 79,
    102-103, 104, 105,
    136, 143
*L. hybrida (L. x intermedia)
    (Lavandin)* 104, 105
L. latifolia (Lavender Spike)
    102, 103, 104-105
L. vera (English Lavender) 102
Lavandin 104, 105
Lavender oil 22-23, 36, 37,
    38, 39, 49, 61, 63, 79,
    102-103, 104, 105,
    114, 116, 126, 136,
    140, 143, 148, 152
  in massage 26, 28, 30, 33
Lavender Spike oil 102, 103,
    104-105
Lemon Balm *see* Melissa oil
Lemon oil 23, 39, 66, 68-69,
    72, 83
  in massage 28
Lemongrass oil 38, 82-83, 84,
    86, 109
  in massage 33
Leptosperum petersonii (Lemon
    Tea Tree) 109
Lime oil 66-67, 68, 72

Mandarin oil 39, 49, 66, 68,
    72-73, 74
  in massage 26, 32
Marjoram oil, Sweet 126-127
massage 24-25
*Matricaria chamomilla (M.
    recutita)* (German
    Chamomile) 36, 37,
    50, 51, 79, 99,
    106-107, 146
Melaleuca alternifolia (Tea
    Tree) 36, 38, 67, 83,
    86, 108-109, 110, 112,
    122, 126, 149

M. leucadendron (M. cajuputi)
    (Cajuput) 38, 59,
    100-111, 113
M. quinquinervia (Niaouli)
    110, 112-113
Melissa officinalis (Melissa,
    Lemon Balm) 114-115
Melissa oil 114-115
menstrual pain 91, 125, 143
Mentha piperita (Peppermint)
    37, 116-117, 119, 130
M. spicata (Spearmint)
    118-119
Moroccan Chamomile oil 51
muscular aches and pains 42,
    100, 110-111, 113,
    120, 123, 133, 140,
    152
Myristca fragrans (Nutmeg)
    120-121
Myrrh oil 36, 56, 76-77, 146
Myrtle oil 37, 38, 122-123
Myrtus communis (Myrtle) 37,
    38, 122-123

nausea 119, 154
Neroli oil 39, 49, 60-61, 62,
    63, 73
  in massage 27
Nerolina oil 113
nervous exhaustion 115, 143
nervous tension 51
Niaouli oil 110, 112-113
Nutmeg oil 120-121

Ocimum basilicum (Basil)
    124-125
O. sanctum (Holy Basil) 124
odor conditioning 23
oily skin 63, 96, 129
Orange Blossom *see* Neroli oil
Orange oil, Sweet 23, 66, 68,
    72, 73, 74-75
Origanum majorana (Sweet
    Marjoram) 126-127
O. vulgare 126
Ormenis mixta (O. multicola)
    (Moroccan Chamomile)
    51

Palmarosa oil 83, 84-85, 86
Patchouli oil 39, 136-137,
    144, 152
Pelargonium x *asperum* 129
P. capitatum 129
P. graveolens (Geranium) 85,
    128-129

P. odoratissimum 129
P. roseum 129
Pepper oil, Black 134-135
  in massage 32
Peppermint oil 22, 23, 37,
    114, 116-117, 118,
    119, 130
  in massage 33
Petitgrain oil 62-63, 66
Pimenta dioica (Allspice) 100
P. racemosa (Indian Bay) 100
Pimpinella anisum (Aniseed)
    79, 130-131
pimples 36, 76, 149
Pine oil 23, 42, 80, 96,
    132-133
  Scotch 133
Pinus pinaster (Pine) 42,
    132-133
P. sylvestris (Scotch Pine) 133
Piper nigrum (Black Pepper)
    134-135
Pogostemon cablin (Patchouli)
    39, 136-137, 152
premenstrual syndrome (PMS)
    47, 51, 143
Pseudotsuga menziesii
    (Douglas Fir) 42

respiratory congestion 130
respiratory infections 42, 47,
    89, 92, 109
rheumatic pain 37, 79
Roman Chamomile oil 39, 50-
    51, 92, 106
Rosa centifolia 139
R. damascena (Rose) 36, 85,
    129, 138-139
Rose oil 21, 23, 27, 36, 52,
    60, 85, 129, 138-139
Rosemary oil 20, 22, 23, 37,
    39, 104, 105, 114,
    126, 140-141, 148
  in massage 28, 32
Rosewood oil 48-49
Rosmarinus officinale
    (Rosemary) 20, 37, 39,
    105, 140-141

Salvia sclarea (Clary Sage)
    142-143
Sandalwood oil 23, 36, 38, 39,
    58, 85, 94, 144-145
  in massage 27, 30
Santalum album (Sandalwood)
    36, 38, 39, 58,
    144-145

S. spicatum 144
Savin oil 96
sexual desire, lack of 55, 150
shaving rash 66-67
shingles 139
shortness of breath 52
sinuses, blocked 89
sleep problems 39, 65, 102
sluggish feeling 154
Spearmint oil 118-119
sprains 92
spritz 74
stress 61, 102, 120, 125
*Styrax benzoin (S.
    paralleloneurus)*
    (Benzoin) 38, 146-147
S. tonkinensis 146
sunburn 102
Sweet Bay *see* Bay Laurel oil

Tea Tree oil 36, 38, 67, 83,
    86, 108-109, 111, 112,
    122, 126, 149
  Lemon Tea Tree oil 109
  in massage 33
thrush 38, 109
Thyme oil 37, 114, 126, 140,
    148-149
Thymus vulgaris (Thyme) 37,
    126, 148-149
tinctures 16
tiredness 72, 83
travel sickness 119
Tulsi 124
Turpentine oil 132

Vanilla oil 150-151
  in massage 32
Vanilla planifolia (V. fragrans)
    (Vanilla) 150-151
V. tahitiensis 150
vegetable oils 17
Vetiver oil 39, 152-153
Vetivera zizanoides (Vetiver)
    39, 152-153

warts 69
wrinkles 49, 52, 76, 85

Yarrow oil 38, 44-45, 90
Ylang ylang oil 23, 39, 54-55
  in massage 30

Zdravetz oil 128
Zingiber officinalis Roscoe
    (Ginger) 58, 93,
    154-155